"Life is a gift, and it offers us the privilege, opportunity, and responsibility to give something back by becoming more."

Tony Robbins

Welcome to the p-i-l-a-t-e-s
Core Stability Ball Instructor Manual

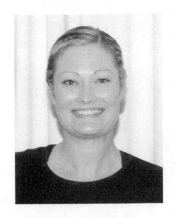

I began learning Pilates as a dancer with knee problems in Melbourne 1991. I moved to London where I undertook my training through Body Control Pilates with Lynne Robinson and Gordon Thomson.

During the 6 years I was teaching in London, I became a Senior Instructor/Examiner and developed workshops and choreographed videos for BCP, lectured at teacher training professional development weekends as well as teaching a variety of clients such as Elizabeth Hurley, Pat Cash, The Wimbledon Football Club, The English National Ballet and The British Olympic Rowing Team.

In 2006 I moved to Asia for a two year teaching contract and began to develop the idea of an on-line Pilates program for Instructors to be able to learn different variations from the mainstream Pilates exercises.

Now back in Australia running my own p-i-l-a-t-e-s studio, I am continuing to develop more programs for Instructors to use as a resource.

The Core Stability Ball is the final manual in the p-i-l-a-t-e-s manual series.

In the p-i-l-a-t-e-s series there are 27 Manuals that include over 1200 exercises.

In this Instructional Manual we offer 76 exercises over 5 Levels for Instructors to learn how to safely and effectively progress your clients using the core stability ball.

Keep an eye out for the new website where you can access video tutorials, webinars and lecture dates for specific courses.

I hope that you find this manual informative and a helpful guide when planning your Core Stability workout for your clients.

Best of luck with your Pilates Career!

Catherine Wilks

Introduction to the Pezzi Ball, Swiss Ball, Fit Ball, Core Ball.

The Core Stability ball, widely known as the "Swiss Ball" around the world was invented in Italy in 1963 by a toy engineer Aqulino Cosani in a plastics factory.

The term "Swiss Ball" was more commonly used after American physical therapists started using ball exercises after witnessing their benefits in Switzerland.

The "Swiss Ball" was used to treat neuromuscular disorders such as MS, cerebral palsy and spinal injuries. Since then, these balls have been known by many different names such as the Fit Ball, Physio Ball, Pilates Ball, Large Ball, Core Ball and Core Stability Ball.

From their initial development in clinical settings, these balls became popular in fitness, personal training and pilates. The reason the these balls became so popular is they allow for a complete multidimensional movement that requires strength, balance and control.

When used with neuro-kinesthetic training, these balls effectively develop core strength, internal balance, stimulate reflexes, improve flexibility and joint range of motion.

We use the balls in a Pilates workout from the basic level of re-training core stability and balance, to an advanced workout requiring an increased level strength, more so than just in a Mat Work session.

The size of the Core Stability Ball can vary, usually in 3 sizes, 55cm, 65cm, and 75cm. Physical therapists suggest using a ball that fits each person's height and leg length is the appropriate way to ensure the best workout is achieved. When sitting a client on the ball ensure the hips are not lower than the knees.

The biggest challenge for all clients using the ball for any Pilates instructor is safety. Unlike the Reformer or Cadillac which are stable, the challenge of the ball is it offers an unstable surface for a challenging workout, offer this piece of equipment to a client who has poor balance, poor core stability and poor strength and you could be in for a bit of a disaster.

The ball is inflatable and usually made out of vinyl or plastic. It is important the client is not wearing any jewellery (sharp rings) that may puncture the ball.

The ball may become weak if exposed to excess sunlight so choose a position In the studio that is out of the way and safe.

Inflatable balls usually require an air pump to fill them up.

Instructions about air pressure are usually provided by the manufacturer. Buy a ball that is good quality for your studio, increases the safety for the client and lasts longer and saves you money.

When used correctly there are many benefits in a Pilates workout:

• it massages the spine increasing disc nutrition

• it increases core strength and stability

• it challenges proprioception

• it challenge the reflexes

• it increases cardiovascular fitness

• it increases flexibility

This manual will offer as a guide for Pilates Instructors, Personal Trainers, Fitness Enthusiasts and Dancers who use the ball to challenge themselves ,and clients with the ball.

It contains 76 exercises from Level 1, Beginner to Level 5, Advanced.

Please ensure that you progress through each level in order to build strength, control and balance. The ball is a fantastic challenge and I hope you enjoy using it for a full body Pilates workout.

Summary of Core Stability Ball Exercises

p-i-l-a-t-e-s
Core Stability Ball - Core Stability - Level 1
Exercise 1 - Single Leg Press

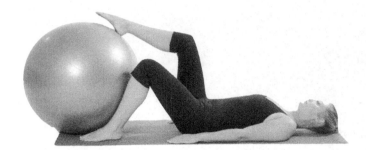

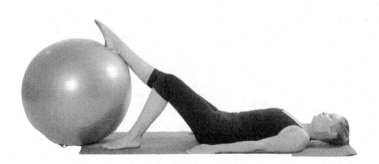

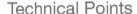

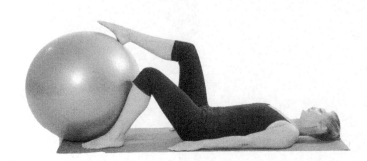

Exercise Focus

This exercise challenges core stability and is a great exercise for clients with back problems.

Start Position

Lying semi-supine on the mat, engage the abdominals and lift the right knee up to the "table top" position, place the right heel on the ball about a half way down the ball, arms relaxed by the side of the body, ensure the pelvis and spine are in neutral.

Exhale to engage the abdominals and slowly roll the ball away from the hip until the right leg is straight.

Inhale and initiating from the hamstrings, roll the ball in one straight line along the mat returning to the start position.

Repeat the exercise 5 times with the right leg, then change to the left leg.

Technical Points

Keep your spine and pelvis in neutral as the leg bends and extends.

Keep the pelvis steady, try not to tilt the pelvis to one side.

Keep the shoulders and neck relaxed.

Try not to press down with too much pressure into the ball with the supporting foot.

Repetitions

8 Single Leg Press Out on the Ball.

Contra-indications

Reduce the range of knee movement for clients with knee pain.

Basic Anatomy

Transversus Abdominus
Oblique Abdominals
Multifidus
Hamstrings
Hip Flexors

p-i-l-a-t-e-s
Core Stability Ball - Core Stability - Level 1
Exercise 2 - Double Leg Press

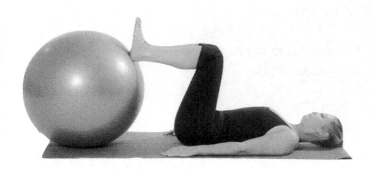

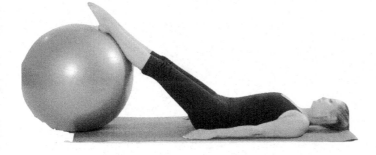

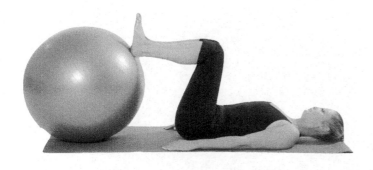

Exercise Focus

This exercise challenges core stability and strengthens the hamstrings.

Start Position

Lying semi-supine on the mat, engage the abdominals and lift the legs one at a time to the "table top" position, place the heels on the ball about a half way down the ball, knees and feet parallel, adducted, arms relaxed by the side of the body, ensure the pelvis and spine are in neutral.

Exhale to engage the abdominals and slowly roll the ball away from the hip until the legs are straight.

Inhale and initiating from the hamstrings, roll the ball in one straight line along the mat returning to the start position.

Technical Points

Keep your spine and pelvis in neutral as the legs straighten and bend.

Keep the pelvis steady, try not to tilt the pelvis anteriorly (arch the back) when rolling the ball away from the hips, or tilt the pelvis posteriorly (tuck the pelvis) when rolling the ball towards the hips.

Keep the shoulders and neck relaxed.

Try not to press down with too much pressure into the ball with the working foot.

Repetitions

8 Double Leg Press Out on the Ball.

Contra-indications

Reduce the range of hip movement for clients with hip replacements.

Avoid with lower back pain.

Basic Anatomy

Transversus Abdominus
Oblique Abdominals
Multifidus
Hamstrings
Hip Flexors

p-i-l-a-t-e-s
Core Stability Ball - Core Stability - Level 1
Exercise 3 - Side Leg Openings

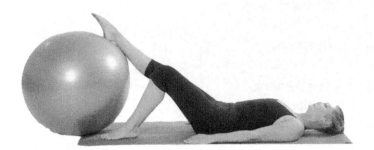

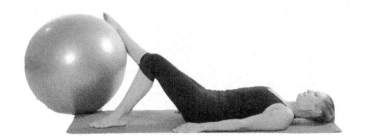

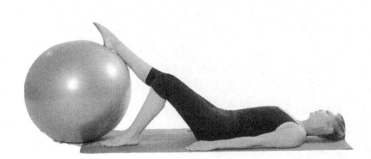

Exercise Focus

This exercise challenges core stability particularly pelvic stability and strengthens the oblique abdominals.

Start Position

Lying semi-supine on the mat, engage the abdominals and raise the right knee towards the chest and place the right heel on the ball with the right leg straight, left foot remains on the mat, pelvis and spine in neutral.

Inhale to prepare and engage the abdominals.

Exhale to slowly roll the ball out to the right only as far as you can control without tilting the pelvis.

Inhale to slowly roll the ball back to the start position.

Repeat the exercise 6 times with the right heel on the ball then change to the left heel.

Technical Points

Keep your spine and pelvis in neutral.

Keep the pelvis steady, try not to tilt the pelvis to one side.

Keep the shoulders and neck relaxed.

Try not to press down with too much pressure into the ball with the working foot.

Repetitions

6 Side Leg Openings each side on the Ball.

Contra-indications

Reduce the range of hip movement for clients with hip replacements.

Basic Anatomy

Transversus Abdominus
Oblique Abdominals
Multifidus
Hamstrings
Hip Flexors

p-i-l-a-t-e-s
Core Stability Ball - Core Stability - Level 1
Exercise 4 - Single Knee Lifts

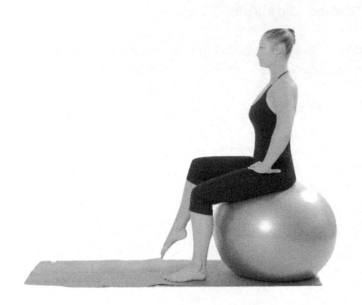

Exercise Focus

This exercise strengthens the deep stabilisers of the spine whilst challenging pelvic and core stability.

Start Position

Sitting on the ball, spine is lengthened, neutral spine and pelvis, hands are placed on the hips, shoulders relaxed, abdominals engaged, feet and knees are hip width apart, ensure that your weight is distributed evenly on both feet.

Inhale to prepare and engage the abdominals.

Exhale to lift your right foot off the floor, folding at the hip, keep the pelvis as stable as possible and try not to shift your weight to one side.

Inhale to lower the right foot to the floor.

Exhale to lift your left foot off the floor, folding at the hip, try to keep your pelvis and spine still and stable.

Inhale to lower the left foot to the floor.

Technical Points

Keep your spine in neutral as you lift your leg.

Use as minimal transference of weight through the feet as possible.

Maintain level hip bones.

Ensure that your ribcage does not move to the opposite side of the leg being raised to counter balance the movement.

Keep your shoulders relaxed.

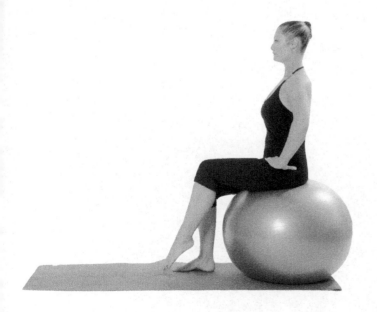

Repetitions

5 leg lifts each side

Contra-indications

Avoid with any back pain, acute disc injuries.

Basic Anatomy

Transversus Abdominus
Oblique Abdominals
Multifidus
Erector Spinae
Illiopsoas
Hip Flexors
Quadriceps

p-i-l-a-t-e-s
Core Stability Ball - Core Stability - Level 1
Exercise 5 - Rotation

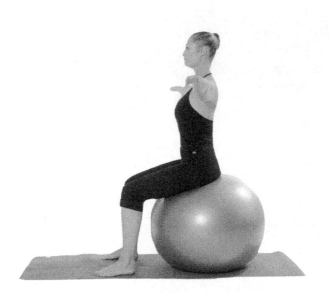

Exercise Focus

This exercise strengthens and stretches deep spinal rotators whilst challenging core and pelvic stability.

Start Position

Sitting on the ball, spine is lengthened, neutral spine and pelvis, arms are extended out to the sides of the body, scapular stabilised and abominals engaged, ensure the weight is even on both feet.

Inhale to prepare.

Exhale to rotate your spine towards the right, ensuring you turn your head first, then sequentially rotating your spine to as far as you can turn without moving your pelvis or feet.

Inhale to return your spine to centre and check your head, ribcage and pelvis all stack in alignment.

Repeat to the other side.

Technical Points

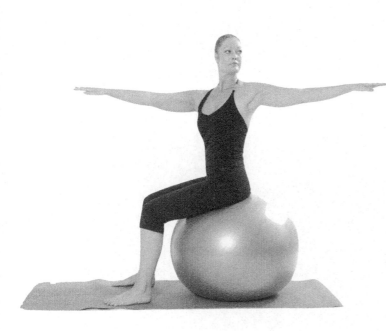

Keep your spine lengthening out through the top of your head as you rotate.

Use as minimal transference of weight through the feet as possible.

Ensure that your ribcage does not shift out of alignment when rotating your spine.

Engage your abdominals throughout the exercise.

Try not to lean backwards.

Keep your shoulders relaxed.

Repetitions

3 rotations to each side.

Contra-indications

Avoid with any back pain, acute disc injuries.

Basic Anatomy

Transversus Abdominis
Multifidus
Deep Spinal Rotores Muscles
Obliques
Erector Spinae
HIp Flexors

p-i-l-a-t-e-s
Core Stability Ball - Core Stability - Level 1
Exercise 6 - Side Bend

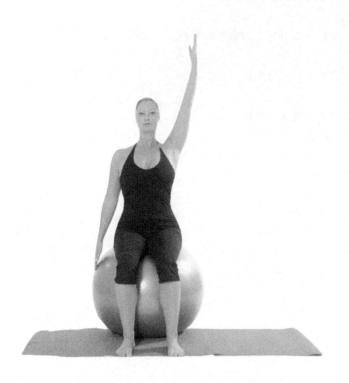

Exercise Focus

This exercise stretches and strengthens side flexors of the body.

Start Position

Sitting on the ball, spine is lengthened, neutral spine and pelvis, one hand placed on your hip, the other arm in raised above the shoulder, scapular stabilised and abominals engaged, ensure that your weight is distributed evenly on both feet.

Inhale to prepare.

Exhale to lift lengthen your spine and side bend to the right, keep your left shoulder blade down the back.

Inhale to return your spine to centre, keeping the pelvis as still and stable on the ball.

Repeat the exercise 5 times side bending to the left, then repeat the exercise 5 times side bending to the right.

Technical Points

Keep your spine lengthening up as you side bend.

Use as minimal transference of weight through the feet as possible.

Ensure that your side bend is from the waistline and not from displacing the ribcage.

Keep your pelvis centered on the ball, try not to lift the opposite hip as you side bend.

Keep your shoulders relaxed.

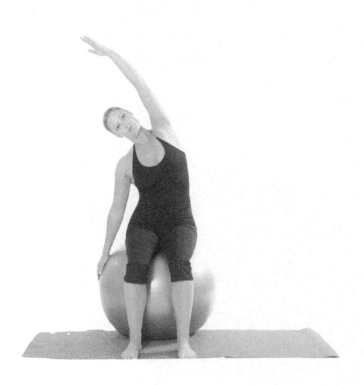

Repetitions

5 side bends to each side.

Contra-indications

Avoid with any back pain, acute disc injuries.

Basic Anatomy

Transversus Abdominis
Obliques
Quadratus Lumborum
Side Flexors of the Spine
Hip Flexors

p-i-l-a-t-e-s
Core Stability Ball - Core Stability - Level 1
Exercise 7 - Bounces Feet Apart

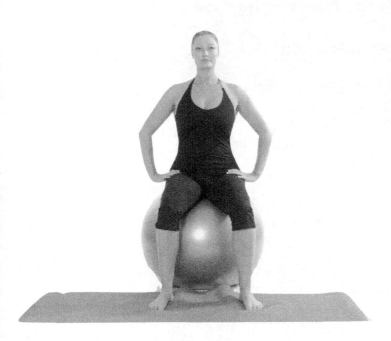

Exercise Focus

This exercise challenges the core stabilisers of the spine and massages the inter-vertabral discs.

Start Position

Sitting on the ball, spine is lengthened, neutral spine and pelvis, hands are on hips, elbows out to the sides, scapular stabilised and abdominals engaged, ensure that your weight is distributed evenly on both feet, feet and knees are hip width apart.

Begin with your feet apart and bounce up and down on the ball, keeping your spine lengthened, try to keep the weight even on your sits bones and feet as you bounce.

Inhale for 2 bounces and then exhale for 2 bounces.

Technical Points

Keep your spine in neutral as you bounce on the ball.

Keep the weight even on both feet as you bounce.

Ensure that your abdominals are engaged and your spine remains centered over the pelvis, be careful not to lean backwards.

Keep your shoulders relaxed.

Repetitions

20 Small Bounces with the feet apart.

Contra-indications

Avoid with any back pain, acute disc injuries.

Basic Anatomy

Transversus Abdominis
Obliques
Multifidus
Erector Spinae
Hamstrings
Gluteals

p-i-l-a-t-e-s
Core Stability Ball - Core Stability - Level 1
Exercise 8 - Bounces In/Out

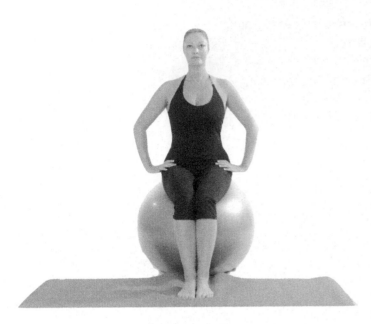

Exercise Focus

This exercise challenges the core stabilisers of the spine and massages the intervertabral discs whilst challenging co-ordination.

Start Position

Sitting on the ball, spine is lengthened, neutral spine and pelvis, hands are on hips, elbows out to the sides, scapular stabilised and abdominals engaged, ensure that your weight is distributed evenly on both feet, feet and knees are hip width apart.

Begin with your feet together and bounce up and down on the ball, keeping your spine lengthened, try to keep the weight even on your sits bones and feet as you bounce.

Inhale for 2 bounces with the feet apart and then exhale for 2 bounces bringing the feet and knees together.

Technical Points

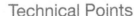

Keep your spine in neutral as you bounce on the ball.

Keep the weight even on both feet as you bounce.

Ensure that your abdominals are engaged and your spine remains centred over the pelvis, be careful not to lean backwards.

Keep your shoulders relaxed.

Maintain a consistent rhythm for 2 bounces in and 2 bounces out.

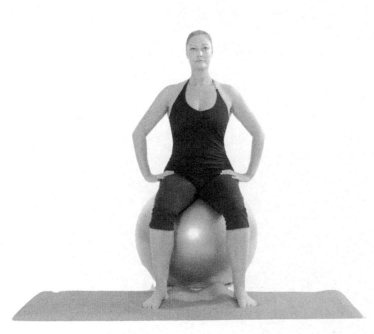

Repetitions

20 Small Bounces (10 times, feet together for 2 bounces, feet apart for 2 bounces).

Contra-indications

Avoid with any back pain, acute disc injuries.

Basic Anatomy

Transversus Abdominis
Obliques
Multifidus
Erector Spinae
Adductors of the Hip
Abductors of the Hip
Hamstrings
Gluteals

p-i-l-a-t-e-s
Core Stability Ball - Pelvic Roll Up - Level 1
Exercise 9 - Knees Bent

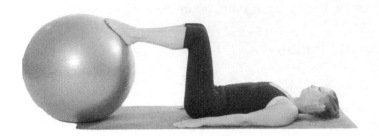

Exercise Focus

This exercise strengthens the hamstrings and gluteals whilst mobilising the spine.

Start Position

Lying on the mat, place the legs on the ball, mid to lower calves on the ball, legs adducted, arms rested by the sides of the body, pelvis and spine in a neutral position.

Inhale to prepare and engage the abdominals.

Exhale to curl the tailbone under and posteriorly tilt the pelvis (tuck the pelvis under) and curl the spine off the mat bone by bone, raise the pelvis off the floor.

Inhale to hold the position, relax the shoulders.

Exhale to segmentally roll the spine back down onto the mat until the pelvis returns to a neutral spine.

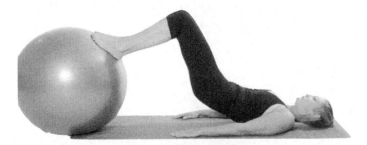

Technical Points

Keep the shoulders, neck and arms relaxed.

Maintain the ball as still and stable as possible.

Keep the legs adducted.

As the pelvis is lifted, try not to raise the pelvis too high and arch the lower back.

Repetitions

5 Pelvic Roll Ups with Bent Knees on the Ball.

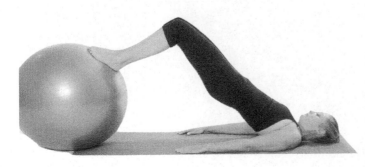

Contra-indications

Avoid with lower back pain or disc injuries.

Avoid with neck pain or whiplash pathology.

Avoid during pregnancy.

Basic Anatomy

Transversus Abdominus
Oblique Abdominals
Rectus Abdominus
Multifidus
Hamstrings
Quadriceps
Illiopsoas
Deep Neck Flexors
Scapula Stabilisers

p-i-l-a-t-e-s
Core Stability Ball - Pelvic Roll Up - Level 2
Exercise 10 - Legs Straight

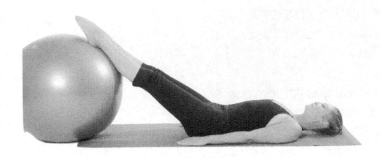

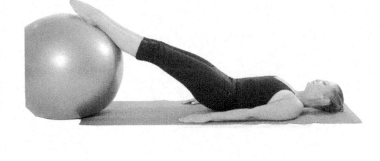

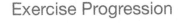

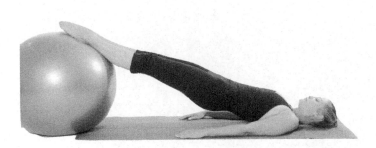

Exercise Focus

This exercise strengthens the hamstrings and gluteals whilst mobilising the spine.

Start Position

Lying on the mat, place the legs on the ball, lower calves and heels on the ball, legs straight and adducted, arms rested by the sides of the body, feet softly pointed.

Inhale to prepare and engage the abdominals.

Exhale to curl the tailbone under and posteriorly tilt the pelvis (tuck the pelvis under) and curl the spine off the mat bone by bone, raise the pelvis off the floor.

Inhale to hold the position, relax the shoulders, keep the ball as still and stable as possible.

Exhale to segmentally roll the spine back down onto the mat until the pelvis returns to a neutral spine.

Exercise Progression

If you are able to roll up and down the spine with the ball still and stable, try raising both arms slightly off the mat to further challenge core stability.

Technical Points

Keep the shoulders, neck and arms relaxed.

Maintain the ball as still and stable as possible.

Keep the legs adducted and straight.

As the pelvis is lifted, try not to raise the pelvis too high and arch the lower back.

Repetitions

5 Pelvic Roll Ups with Straight Legs on the Ball.

Contra-indications

Avoid with lower back pain or disc injuries.

Avoid with neck pain or whiplash pathology.

Avoid during pregnancy.

Basic Anatomy

Transversus Abdominus
Oblique Abdominals
Rectus Abdominus
Multifidus
Hamstrings
Quadriceps
Illiopsoas
Deep Neck Flexors
Scapula Stabilisers

p-i-l-a-t-e-s
Core Stability Ball - Single Leg Stretch - Level 1
Exercise 11 - Bicycle

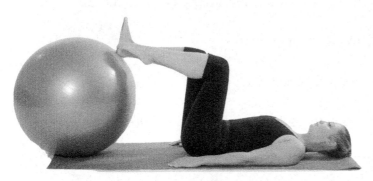

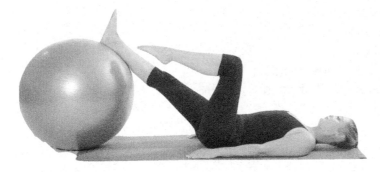

Exercise Focus

This exercise challenges core stability whilst strengthening the hamstrings and hip flexors.

Start Position

Lying on the mat, place the feet on the ball, feet and knees hip width apart, knees bent at a 90° over the hips, pelvis and spine in a neutral position, arms rested by the sides of the body.

Inhale to prepare and engage the abdominals.

Exhale to keep the left knee still and roll the right heel away from the hip until the right leg is straight.

Inhale to roll the right heel back in towards the body, keeping the pelvis and spine in a neutral position.

Repeat the exercise 5 times with the right heel on the ball, then repeat the exercise 5 times with the left heel on the ball.

Technical Points

Maintain the pelvis and spine in neutral as the leg fully extends away from the hip, try not to allow the lumbar lordosis to increase.

Keep the neck, shoulders and arms relaxed by the side of the body and isolate the movement in the legs and abdominals.

Keep the navel drawn gently back towards the spine throughout the entire exercise.

Try to roll the ball in and out in one straight line, keep the knee in line with the 2nd metatarsal.

Repetitions

10 Single Leg Stretch Bicycle on the Ball.

Contra-indications

Avoid with lower back pain.

Avoid during pregnancy.

Basic Anatomy

Transversus Abdominus
Oblique Abdominals
Multifidus
Hamstrings
Quadriceps
Hip Flexors
Scapula Stabilisers

p-i-l-a-t-e-s
Core Stability Ball - Side To Side - Level 1
Exercise 12 - Legs On The Ball

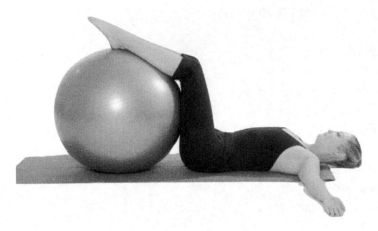

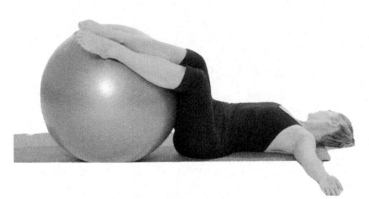

Exercise Focus

This exercise strengthens the oblique abdominal muscles whilst stretching and strengthening the rotores muscles of the spine.

Start Position

Lying on the semi-supine on the mat, place both legs over the ball, arms are extended to the sides of the body slightly below shoulder height, palms to the ceiling.

Inhale to engage the abdominals and roll the ball to the right, keep the shoulder blades in contact with the mat.

Exhale to use the abdominals to return the ball to the centre.

Inhale to roll the ball to the left side, keep the shoulder blades in contact with the mat.

Exhale to return the ball to the centre.

Technical Points

Keep the shoulder blades drawing down the back.

Keep the navel drawn gently back towards the spine throughout the entire exercise.

Keep the opposite shoulder blade in contact with the mat as the legs roll to the side.

Try not to posteriorly tilt the pelvis under as the legs return the ball to the centre.

Repetitions

5 Side to Side with Legs on the Ball.

Contra-indications

Avoid with lower back pain or disc injuries.

Avoid with neck pain or pathology such as whiplash or osteoarthritis.

Avoid during pregnancy.

Basic Anatomy

Transversus Abdominus
Oblique Abdominals
Multifidus
Hip Flexors
Spinal Rotores
Scapula Stabilisers
Arm Extensors

p-i-l-a-t-e-s
Core Stability Ball - Knee Bends - Level 1
Exercise 13 - Parallel

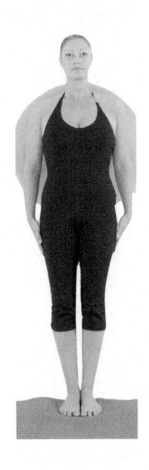

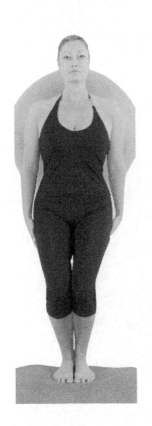

Exercise Focus

This exercise strengthens the quadriceps and calves whilst challenging spinal alignment.

Start Position

Standing against the wall, place the ball between the shoulder blades, lean on the ball, standing with the feet comfortably forward, feet and legs together, spine and pelvis in a neutral position, arms by the side of the body.

Inhale to engage the abdominals and bend the knees directly over the 2nd metatarsals, keep the pelvis in neutral.

Exhale to extend the legs.

Technical Points

Try not to allow the pelvis to arch in the lumbar area and follow the ball, try to bend from the knees and keep the tailbone dropping directly to the floor.

Keep the arms relaxed by the sides of the body.

Keep the spine lengthened.

Keep the abdominals gently drawn back towards the spine.

Ensure the weight is evenly distributed on both feet.

When bending the knees maintain the heels in contact with the floor.

Repetitions

10 Knee Bends in Parallel with the Ball.

Contra-indications

Avoid with knee pain or hip pain.

Basic Anatomy

Transversus Abdominus
Oblique Abdominals
Multifidus
Quadriceps
Erector Spinae
Gluteus Medius
Gluteus Maximus
Hip Flexors
Gastrocnemius
Soleus
Foot Flexors and Extensors

p-i-l-a-t-e-s
Core Stability Ball - Knee Bends - Level 1
Exercise 14 - Pilates "V Position

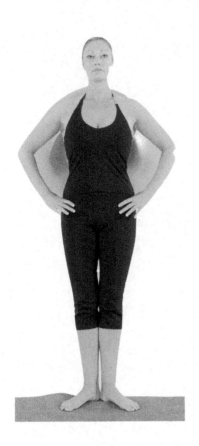

Exercise Focus

This exercise strengthens the lateral rotators of the pelvis and hip flexors and challenges spinal alignment.

Start Position

Standing against the wall, place the ball between the shoulder blades, lean on the ball, standing with the feet comfortably forward, feet and legs turned out, heels together toes apart in the Pilates "V" position, spine and pelvis in a neutral position, arms by the side of the body.

Inhale to engage the abdominals and bend the knees directly over the 2nd metatarsals, knees apart, keep the pelvis in neutral.

Exhale to straighten the legs drawing the inner thighs together.

Technical Points

Try not to allow the pelvis to arch in the lumbar area and follow the ball, try to bend from the knees and keep the tailbone dropping directly to the floor.

Keep the arms relaxed by the sides of the body.

Keep the spine lengthened.

Keep the abdominals gently drawn back towards the spine.

Ensure the weight is evenly distributed on both feet.

When bending the knees maintain the heels in contact with the floor.

Repetitions

10 Knee Bends in the Pilates "V" Position with the Ball.

Contra-indications

Avoid with knee pain or hip pain.

Basic Anatomy

Transversus Abdominus
Oblique Abdominals
Multifidus
Quadriceps
Adductors
Erector Spinae
Gluteus Maximus
Gluteus Medius
Lateral Rotators of the Hips
Hip Flexors
Gastrocnemius
Soleus
Foot Flexors and Extensors

p-i-l-a-t-e-s
Core Stability Ball - Knee Bends - Level 1
Exercise 15 - Feet Wide

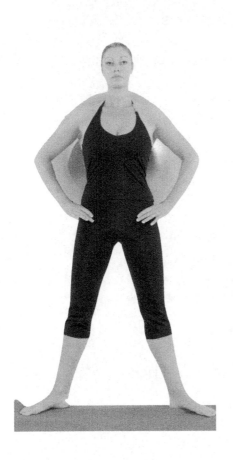

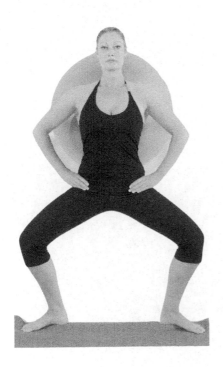

Exercise Focus

This exercise strengthens the lateral rotators, quadriceps and adductors of the legs whilst challenging spinal alignment.

Start Position

Standing against the wall, place the ball between the shoulder blades, lean on the ball, standing with the feet comfortably forward, feet and knees wide apart, slightly laterally rotated from the hips, spine and pelvis in a neutral position, arms by the side of the body.

Inhale to engage the abdominals and bend the knees directly over the 2nd metatarsals, keep the pelvis in neutral.

Exhale to extend the legs, lift the knee caps to use the quadriceps as the legs fully straighten.

Technical Points

Try not to allow the pelvis to arch in the lumbar area and follow the ball, try to bend from the knees and keep the tailbone dropping directly to the floor.

Keep the arms relaxed by the sides of the body.

Keep the spine lengthened.

Keep the abdominals gently drawn back towards the spine.

Ensure the weight is evenly distributed on both feet.

When bending the knees maintain the heels in contact with the floor.

Repetitions

10 Knee Bends with Feet Wide with the Ball.

Contra-indications

Avoid with knee pain or hip pain.

Basic Anatomy

Transversus Abdominus
Oblique Abdominals
Multifidus
Quadriceps
Erector Spinae
Adductors
Lateral Rotators of the Hip
Gluteus Medius
Gluteus Maximus
Hip Flexors
Gastrocnemius
Soleus
Foot Flexors and Extensors

p-i-l-a-t-e-s
Core Stability Ball - Lunges - Level 1
Exercise 16 - Forward

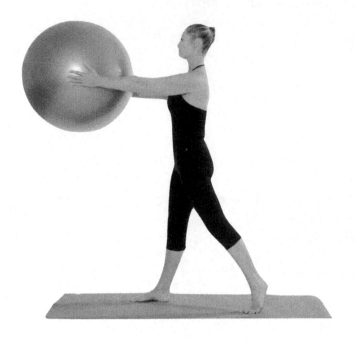

Exercise Focus

This exercise strengthens the gluteals, quadriceps and hamstrings whilst challenging balance and core stability.

Start Position

Standing on the mat, hold the ball in the hands, arms straight in front of the shoulders, place the right foot forward in line with the right hip joint, place the left foot behind the left hip, on the ball of the foot, pelvis in neutral, feet and legs parallel.

Inhale to engage the abdominals and bend both knees keeping most of the weight distribution on the right foot, maintain the arms in front of the body.

Exhale to straighten the legs, maintain the arms at shoulder height.

Inhale to bend the knees directly over the 2nd metatarsal, most of the weight is on the right foot.

Exhale to engage the abdominals and straighten the right leg.

Repeat the exercise 10 Lunges Forward with the right leg in front, then 10 with the left foot forward.

Technical Points

Keep the spine lengthened.

Try not to allow the pelvis to arch in the lumbar area and follow the ball, try to bend from the knees and keep the tailbone dropping directly to the floor.

Keep the abdominals gently drawn back towards the spine.

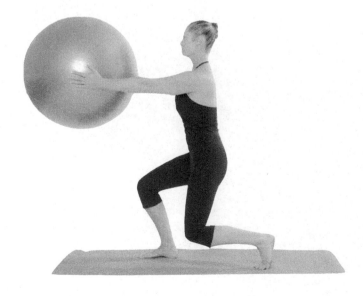

Ensure the pelvis remains level, try not to hike one side of the pelvis up.

Keep the arms in line with the shoulders when performing the exercise.

Repetitions

10 Lunges Forward with the Ball.

Contra-indications

Avoid with knee pain or hip pain.

Basic Anatomy

Transversus Abdominus
Oblique Abdominals
Multifidus
Erector Spinae
Quadriceps
Hamstrings
Gluteus Medius
Gluteus Maximus
Hip Flexors
Gastrocnemius
Soleus
Foot Flexors and Extensors

p-i-l-a-t-e-s
Core Stability Ball - Hip Flexor Stretch - Level 1
Exercise 17 - Forward

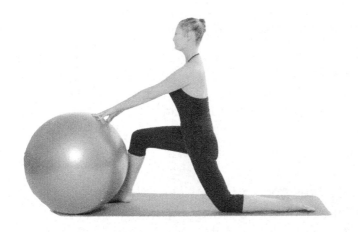

Exercise Focus

This exercise stretches the quadriceps and hip flexors.

Start Position

Kneeling on the mat, place the ball to the right side of the body, place the right foot forward of the right hip, legs parallel, hip width apart, rest the right hand on the ball for support.

Inhale to prepare and engage the abdominals.

Exhale to slowly lean forward taking the weight onto the front leg stretching the left hip flexor.

Ensure when stretching the left leg, the right knee joint is behind the right foot to avoid compressing the knee, hold the stretch for 5 slow deep breaths.

Inhale to slowly press back through the right foot and return the body to the start position.

Technical Points

Keep the spine and pelvis in neutral.

Keep the spine lengthened.

Try not to drop the lower back when extending the legs away from the hips.

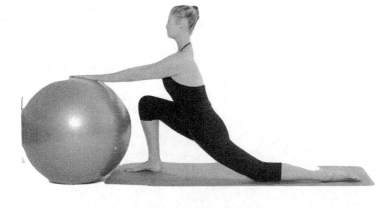

Try not to collapse the shoulder blades together, keep the scapula still and isolate the press in and out from the arms only.

Visualise a strip of tape along the mat, roll the ball along the line.

Keep the abdominals gently drawn back towards the spine.

Ensure the weight is evenly distributed on both arms.

Repetitions

2 Hip Flexor Stretches each leg with the Ball.

Contra-indications

Avoid with knee pain.

Avoid with groin pain.

Avoid with lower back pain.

Basic Anatomy

Transversus Abdominus
Oblique Abdominals
Multifidus
Erector Spinae
HIp Flexors
Illiopsoas
Quadriceps

p-i-l-a-t-e-s
Core Stability Ball - Hip Flexor Stretch - Level 1
Exercise 18 - Hip Flexor/Adductor

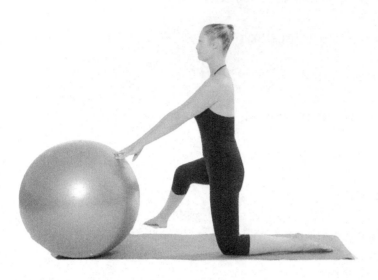

Exercise Focus

This exercise stretches the quadriceps, hip flexors and adductors.

Start Position

Kneeling on the mat, place the ball to the right side of the body, place the left foot forward of the hip 45° to the left hip joint, left leg slightly turned out from the hip, right leg parallel, hip width apart, rest the right hand on the ball for support.

Inhale to prepare and engage the abdominals.

Exhale to slowly lean forward taking the weight onto the front leg stretching the right hip flexor, adductors and pectineus.

Ensure when stretching the right leg, the left knee joint is behind the left foot to avoid compressing the knee, hold the stretch for 5 slow deep breaths.

Inhale to slowly press back through the left foot and return the body to the start position.

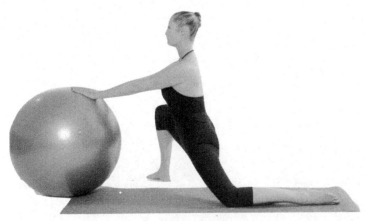
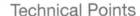

Technical Points

Keep the hips square to the front, do not twist the hips to face the front leg that is stretching.

Keep the abdominals gently drawn back towards the spine.

Repetitions

2 Hip Flexor/Adductor Stretches each leg with the Ball.

Contra-indications

Avoid with knee pain.

Avoid with groin pain.

Avoid with lower back pain.

Basic Anatomy

Transversus Abdominus
Oblique Abdominals
Multifidus
Erector Spinae
HIp Flexors
Illiopsoas
Adductors
Pectineus
Quadriceps

p-i-l-a-t-e-s
Core Stability Ball - Adductor Stretch - Level 1
Exercise 19 - Adductor Stretch

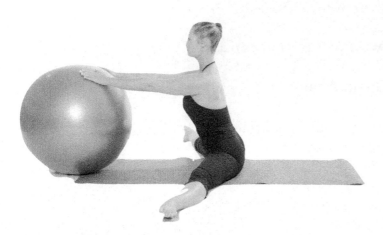

Exercise Focus

This exercise stretches the hamstrings and hip adductors.

Start Position

Sitting on the mat, place the ball between the legs, legs are open wide at the hips, sitting with a neutral spine and pelvis, place the hands on top of the ball.

Inhale to prepare and engage the abdominals.

Exhale to slowly lean forward into the stretch and slowly roll the ball away from the body keeping the arms straight.

Hold the stretch for 5 deep breaths, try not to allow the feet to roll inwards.

Inhale to slowly roll the ball towards the body and roll up out of the stretch

Technical Points

Keep the spine lengthened.

Keep the abdominals gently drawn back towards the spine.

Ensure the weight is evenly distributed on both sits bones.

Try not to allow the legs to roll inwards.

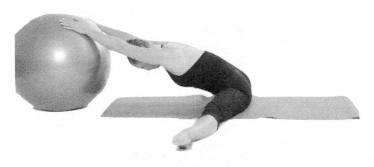

Repetitions

2 Adductor Stretches with the Ball.

Contra-indications

Avoid with knee pain.

Avoid with groin pain.

Avoid with lower back pain.

Basic Anatomy

Transversus Abdominus
Oblique Abdominals
Multifidus
Erector Spinae
Hip Flexors
Adductors
Hamstrings
Illiopsoas
Quadriceps

p-i-l-a-t-e-s
Core Stability Ball - Core Stability - Level 2
Exercise 20 - Single Leg Hop

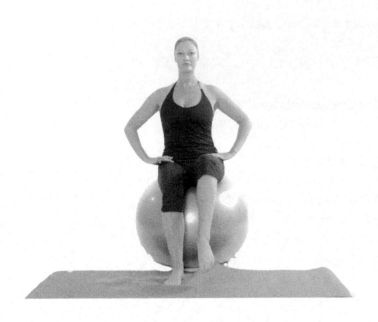

Exercise Focus

This exercise challenges the core stabilisers of the spine and abdominals, enhances neuromuscular co-ordination.

Start Position

Sitting on the ball, spine is lengthened, neutral spine and pelvis, hands are on hips, elbows out to the sides, scapular stabilised and abdominals engaged, ensure that your weight is distributed evenly though the feet, feet and knees are hip width apart.

Raise your right foot off the floor, folding at your hip joint, keep your ribcage centred over your pelvis and spine lengthened.

Inhale and hop on your left leg for 2 hops, keeping your right knee lifted.

Exhale to change legs changing the weight to the right leg and hop on the right leg for 2 hops, keep your left knee lifted.

Continue to alternate legs hopping 2 times on each side.

Technical Points

Keep your spine in neutral as you bounce on the ball.

Keep the weight even on both feet as you bounce.

Ensure that your abdominals are engaged and your spine remains centered over the pelvis, be careful not to lean backwards.

Keep the knee of the leg raised in line with your hip.

Keep your shoulders relaxed.

Repetitions

20 Hops.

Contra-indications

Avoid with any back pain, acute disc injuries.

Basic Anatomy

Transversus Abdominis
Multifidus
Obliques
Hip Flexors
Quadriceps
Hamstrings
Calves
Gluteals

p-i-l-a-t-e-s
Core Stability Ball - Core Stability - Level 2
Exercise 21 - Jogging

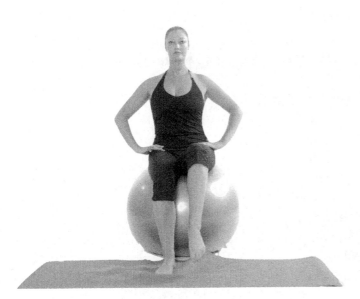

Exercise Focus

This exercise challenges the core stabilisers of the spine and abdominals. Its requires a great deal of co-ordination and control to keep centred on the ball.

Start Position

Sitting on the ball, spine is lengthened, neutral spine and pelvis, hands are on hips, elbows out to the sides, scapular stabilised and abdominals engaged, ensure that your weight is distributed evenly on both feet, feet hip width apart.

Raise your right foot off the floor, folding at your hip joint, keep your ribcage centred over your pelvis and spine lengthened.

Inhale to hop on to the right foot and then changing to hop onto the left foot, continue alternating from one leg to the other, inhale for 2 jogs, then exhale for 2 jogs.

Technical Points

Keep your spine in neutral as you bounce on the ball.

Ensure that your abdominals are engaged.

Keep your spine centered over the pelvis, be careful not to lean backwards.

Keep your shoulders relaxed.

Try not to displace the ribcage to one side as you lift the leg from the hip.

Repetitions

20 small jogs alternating legs.

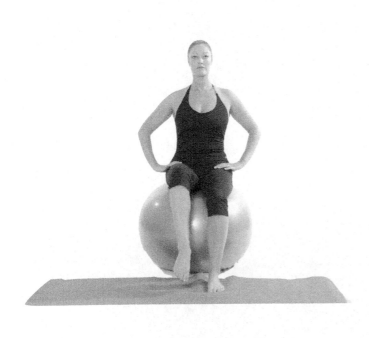

Contra-indications

Avoid with any back pain, acute disc injuries.

Basic Anatomy

Transversus Abdominis
Multifidus
Obliques
Erector Spinae
Illiopsoas
Hip Flexors
Quadriceps
Hamstrings
Gluteals
Calves

p-i-l-a-t-e-s
Core Stability Ball - Core Stability - Level 2
Exercise 22 - Prone Arm/Leg Lifts

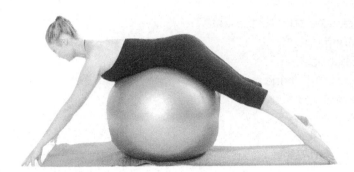

Exercise Focus

This exercise strengthens the spine extensors, hamstrings and mid back stabilisers whilst challenging balance and co-ordination.

Start Position

Lying prone on the ball, place the ball comfortably under the abdomen, arms straight forward, tips of the fingers touching the floor, just wider than shoulder width apart, tips of the toes touching the floor, just wider than hip width apart, distribute the body weight evenly between all 4 points of contact with the floor.

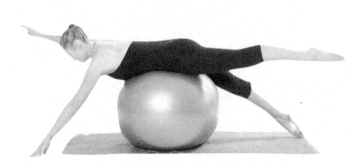

Inhale to prepare and engage the abdominals.

Exhale to stabilise the scapula and raise the right hand and left foot off the floor simultaneously whilst maintaining stillness on the ball.

Inhale to lower the right hand and left foot to the mat.

Exhale to raise the left hand and right foot off the mat, keep stable on the ball.

Inhale to lower the opposite arm and leg.

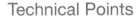

Technical Points

Maintain the abdominals on the lift and lowering of the arm and leg.

The upper body will lift slightly as the arm and leg is lifted, do not increase the lumbar lordosis.

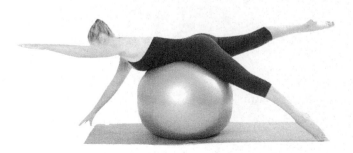

Keep the leg straight when lifting.

Maintain the shoulder blades down the back on both the lifting and lowering.

Try not to twist the body to one side.

Repetitions

6 Opposite Arm and Leg Lifts Prone on the ball.

Contra-indications

Avoid with any back pain.

Avoid with neck pain.

Basic Anatomy

Transversus Abdominis
Multifidus
Erector Spinae
Gluteus Maximus
Hamstrings
Lower/Mid Trapezius

p-i-l-a-t-e-s
Core Stability Ball - Core Stability - Level 2
Exercise 23 - Four Corner Touch

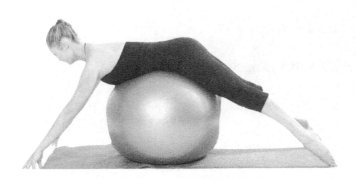

Exercise Focus

This exercise requires concentration, control and balance, it challenges the neuromuscular control of the arms and legs.

Start Position

Lying prone on the ball, place the ball comfortably under the abdomen, arms forward, slightly bent at the elbows, tips of the fingers touching the floor, just wider than shoulder width apart, tips of the toes touching the floor, just wider than hip width apart, legs slightly bent, distribute the body weight evenly between all 4 points of contact with the floor.

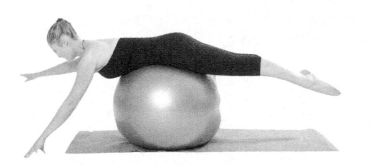

Inhale to prepare and engage the abdominals.

Exhale to stabilse the scapula and roll the ball slightly to the right place all the weight on the right tips of the fingers, raise the other 3 points of contact off the floor.

Inhale to slowly transfer the weight to the left hand, keeping 3 points of contact off the floor at all times.

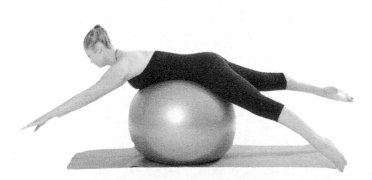

Exhale to transfer the weight to the left foot, maintain a slow controlled movement.

Inhale to transfer the weight to the right foot.

Repeat the exercise 2 times clockwise then 2 times anti-clockwise.

Technical Points

Maintain the abdominals on the transference of weight.

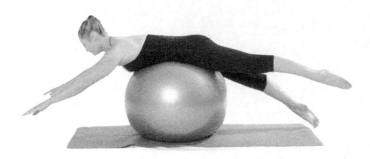
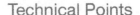

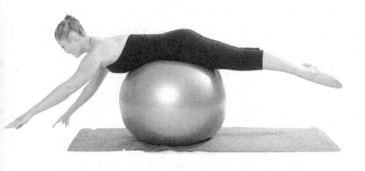

Repetitions

2 Sets of Four Corner Touch in each direction on the ball.

Contra-indications

Avoid with any back pain.

Avoid with neck pain.

Basic Anatomy

Transversus Abdominis
Multifidus
Erector Spinae
Gluteus Maximus
Hamstrings
Lower/Mid Trapezius

p-i-l-a-t-e-s
Core Stability Ball - Walk Downs - Level 2
Exercise 24 - Forward

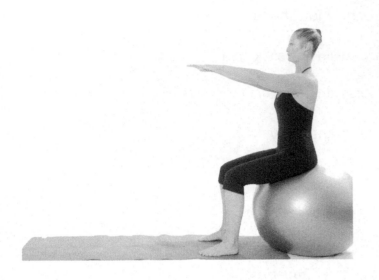

Exercise Focus

This exercise mobilises the spine and strengthens the abdominals whilst challenging co-ordination and control.

Start Position

Sitting on the ball, feet and knees hip width apart, arms raised forward at shoulder height, scapula stabilised, pelvis and spine in a neutral position.

Inhale to prepare and engage the abdominals.

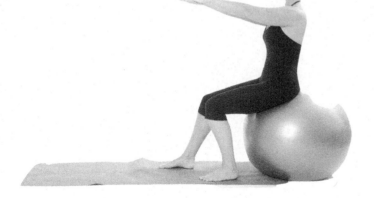

Exhale to curl the tailbone under and roll the spine down onto the ball with control whilst simultaneously walking the feet forwards, walk the feet forwards until your head, neck and shoulders are comfortably placed onto the ball, arms will be directly above the shoulders.

Inhale to hold the position, keep lifting the pelvis and engage the buttocks.

Exhale to engage the abdominals and press through the feet whilst simultaneously drawing the chin towards the chest and roll the spine back up to a sitting position.

Technical Points

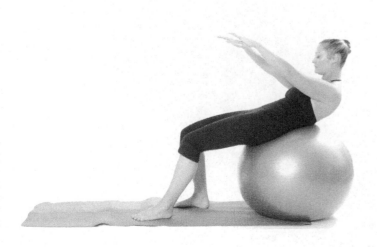

Keep the rolling action down and up off the ball smooth and controlled.

Use a non slip mat on the floor if necessary.

Keep the pelvis lifted when the head, neck and shoulders are on the ball.

Maintain the scapula stability at all times.

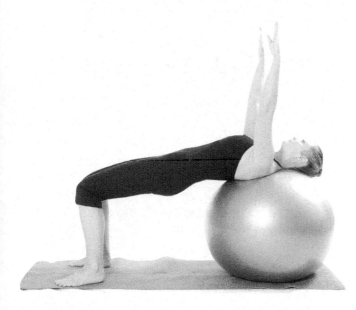

Repetitions

5 Walk Downs on the Ball.

Contra-indications

Avoid with lower back pain or disc injuries.

Avoid with neck pain or whiplash pathology.

Avoid during pregnancy.

Basic Anatomy

Transversus Abdominus
Oblique Abdominals
Rectus Abdominus
Multifidus
Hamstrings
Quadriceps
Illiopsoas
Deep Neck Flexors
Scapula Stabilisers

p-i-l-a-t-e-s
Core Stability Ball - Abdominal Curls - Level 2
Exercise 25 - Forward

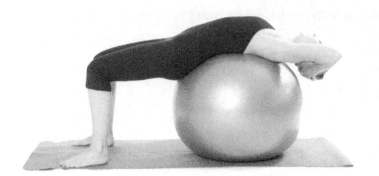

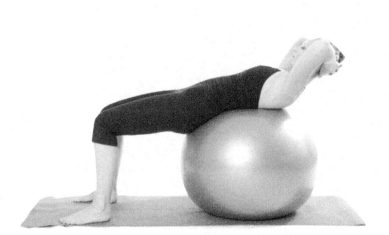

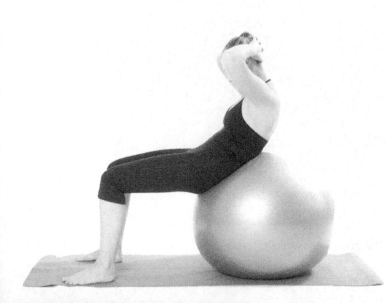

Exercise Focus

This exercise mobilises the spine and strengthens the abdominals.

Start Position

Sitting on the ball, feet and knees hip width apart, arms raised forward at shoulder height, scapula stabilised, pelvis and spine in a neutral position.

Inhale to prepare and engage the abdominals.

Exhale to curl the tailbone under and roll the spine down onto the ball with control whilst simultaneously walking the feet forwards, walk the feet forwards until your head, tailbone is just off the ball, shoulders are comfortably placed onto the ball, interlace the hands behind the head and elbows open in front of the shoulders.

Inhale to extend the spine over the ball as far back as comfortable.

Exhale to curl the upper spine forwards starting from the small nod of the head, curl the head, neck, shoulders forward maintaining a stable pelvis, try not to curl the tailbone under.

Inhale to extend the spine over the ball.

Repeat the abdominal curls for 10 forward, then,

Exhale to engage the abdominals and press through the feet whilst simultaneously drawing the chin towards the chest and roll the spine back up to a sitting position.

Technical Points

Keep the rolling action down and up off the ball smooth and controlled.

Keep the elbows forwards in the peripheral vision when curling and extending the spine.

Keep the eye focus on the abdominals when curling forward, try not to extend the neck and look up to the ceiling.

Try not to arch the lumbar spine when curling back over the ball.

Use a non slip mat on the floor if necessary.

Maintain the scapula stability at all times.

Repetitions

10 Abdominal Curls Forward on the Ball.

Contra-indications

Avoid with lower back pain or disc injuries.

Avoid with neck pain or whiplash pathology.

Avoid during pregnancy.

Basic Anatomy

Transversus Abdominus
Oblique Abdominals
Rectus Abdominus
Multifidus
Hamstrings
Quadriceps
Illiopsoas
Deep Neck Flexors
Scapula Stabilisers

p-i-l-a-t-e-s
Core Stability Ball - Abdominal Curls - Level 2
Exercise 26 - Oblique

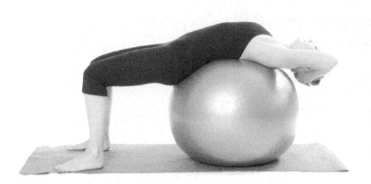

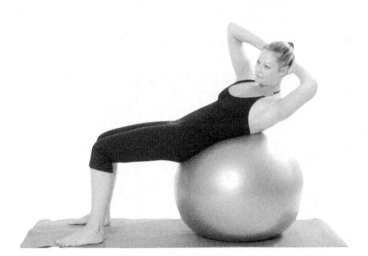

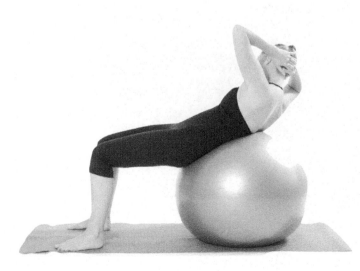

Exercise Focus

This exercise mobilises the spine and strengthens the oblique abdominals.

Start Position

Sitting on the ball, feet and knees hip width apart, arms raised forward at shoulder height, scapula stabilised, pelvis and spine in a neutral position.

Inhale to prepare and engage the abdominals.

Exhale to curl the tailbone under and roll the spine down onto the ball with control whilst simultaneously walking the feet forwards, walk the feet forwards until your head, tailbone is just off the ball, shoulders are comfortably placed onto the ball, interlace the hands behind the head and elbows open in front of the shoulders.

Inhale to extend the spine over the ball as far back as comfortable.

Exhale to curl the upper spine forwards starting from the small nod of the head, curl the head, neck, shoulders forward maintaining a stable pelvis, try not to curl the tailbone under, curl towards the right shoulder blade, the left shoulder blade will come off the ball.

Inhale to extend the spine over the ball returning the spine and shoulders to the centre.

Exhale to curl the upper spine and shoulders forward onto the left shoulder blade, maintain a still and stable pelvis, the right shoulder blade will come off the ball.

Inhale to extend the spine backwards over the ball returning the spine and shoulders to the centre.

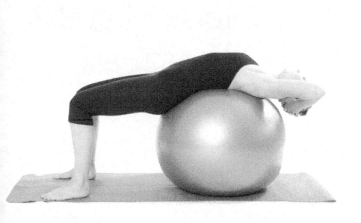

Repeat the exercise 5 times to each side, then, Exhale to engage the abdominals and press through the feet whilst simultaneously drawing the chin towards the chest and roll the spine back up to a sitting position.

Technical Points

Keep the rolling action down and up off the ball smooth and controlled.

Keep the elbows forwards in the peripheral vision when curling and extending the spine.

Keep the eye focus on the abdominals when curling forward, try not to extend the neck and look up to the ceiling.

Try not to arch the lumbar spine when curling back over the ball.

Use a non slip mat on the floor if necessary.

Maintain the scapula stability at all times.

Repetitions

5 Abdominal Curls Oblique to each side on the Ball.

Contra-indications

Avoid with lower back pain or disc injuries.

Avoid with neck pain or whiplash pathology.

Avoid during pregnancy.

Basic Anatomy

Transversus Abdominus
Oblique Abdominals
Rectus Abdominus
Multifidus
Hamstrings
Quadriceps
Illiopsoas
Deep Neck Flexors
Scapula Stabilisers

p-i-l-a-t-e-s
Core Stability Ball - Single Leg Circles - Level 2
Exercise 27 - Pelvis Down

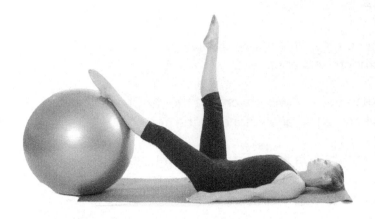

Exercise Focus

This exercise challenges pelvic stability and alignment whilst strengthening the quadriceps and hip flexors of the leg.

Start Position

Lying on the mat, place the feet hip width apart, pelvis and spine in a neutral position, arms rested by the sides of the body, place the ball under the right heel.

Inhale to prepare and engage the abdominals.

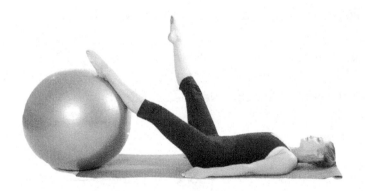

Exhale to roll the right heel away from the hip until the right leg is straight, raise the left leg into the air as high into the air as possible keeping the tailbone on the mat.

Inhale to prepare and engage the abdominals.

Exhale to maintain both legs straight, circle the left leg outwards for 8 small circles, inhaling for 2 circles, exhaling for 2 small circles, keep the ball still and stable.

Inhale to circle the left leg inwards for 8 small circles, inhaling for 2 small circles, then exhaling for 2 circles.

Inhale to lower the left leg down and place the left heel on the ball.

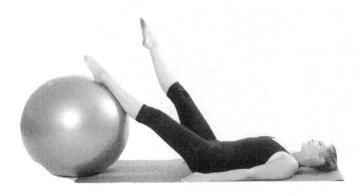

Exhale to raise the right heel off the ball into the air, raise the right leg as high as possible without losing the neutral pelvis.

Inhale as you circle the right leg outwards for 8 small circles, inhaling for 2 circles, exhaling for 2 circles, maintain as still and stable pelvis.

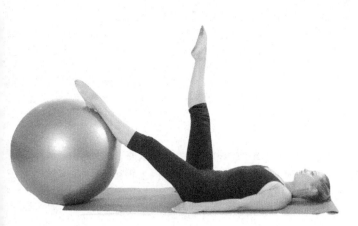

Exhale to circle the right legs inwards for 8 small circles, inhaling for 2 small circles, exhaling for 2 circles.

To finish lower the right leg down and place the right heel onto the ball.

Technical Points

Keep the shoulders relaxed throughout the exercise.

Maintain the ball as still and stable as possible as the working leg is circling.

Keep the legs straight and ensure the tailbone remains on the mat.

Maintain a still and stable pelvis as the leg circles around.

Repetitions

2 Sets of 8 Small Circles each direction with the Pelvis Down on the Ball.

Contra-indications

Avoid with lower back pain or disc injuries.

Avoid with neck pain or whiplash pathology.

Avoid during pregnancy.

Basic Anatomy

Transversus Abdominus
Oblique Abdominals
Multifidus
Hamstrings
Quadriceps
Illiopsoas
Scapula Stabilisers

p-i-l-a-t-e-s
Core Stability Ball - Side To Side - Level 2
Exercise 28 - Feet Up

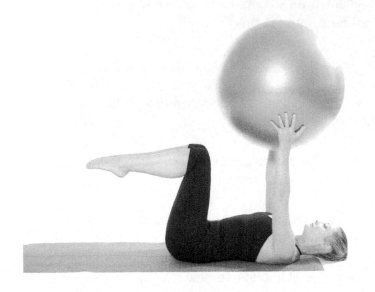

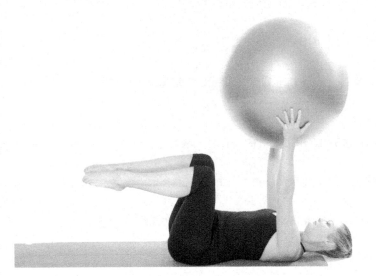

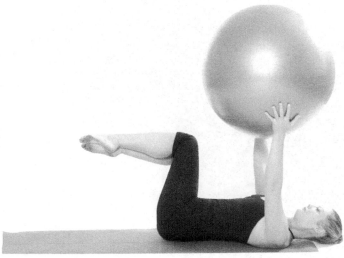

Exercise Focus

This exercise strengthens the oblique abdominals whilst strengthening and stretching the spinal rotores muscles.

Start Position

Lying on the semi-supine on the mat, place the ball in the hands, arms are extended towards the ceiling above the shoulders, legs are lifted one at a time to the "table top" position, knees and feet are adducted, feet softly pointed.

Inhale to engage the abdominals take both legs over to the right, keep the arms still directly above the shoulders, the rotation is purely from the spine and pelvis.

Exhale to use the abdominals to return the legs to the centre.

Inhale to roll onto the left side of the pelvis, keep the shoulder blades in contact with the mat and knees and feet together.

Exhale to use the abdominals and return the legs to the centre.

Technical Points

Keep the shoulder blades in contact with the floor.

Try not to hip hike the pelvis on one side as the legs are taken to the side.

Keep the navel drawn gently back towards the spine throughout the entire exercise.

Keep the opposite shoulder blade in contact with the mat as the legs roll to the side.

Try not to posteriorly tilt the pelvis under as the legs return the ball to the centre.

Repetitions

5 Side to Side with Legs Up with the Ball.

Contra-indications

Avoid with lower back pain or disc injuries.

Avoid with neck pain or pathology such as whiplash or osteoarthritis.

Avoid during pregnancy.

Basic Anatomy

Transversus Abdominus
Oblique Abdominals
Multifidus
Hip Flexors
Spinal Rotores
Scapula Stabilisers
Arm Extensors

p-i-l-a-t-e-s
Core Stability Ball - Knee Bends - Level 2
Exercise 29 - Single Leg

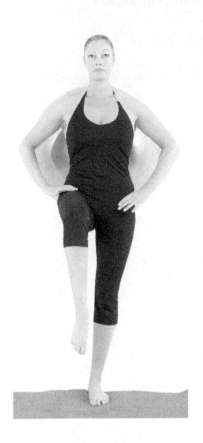

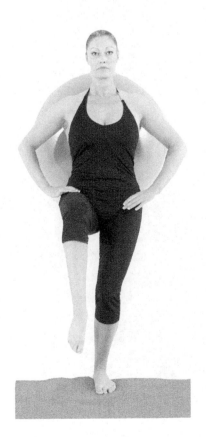

Exercise Focus

This exercise strengthens pelvic and core stability whilst challenging balance and proprioception.

Start Position

Standing against the wall, place the ball between the shoulder blades, lean on the ball, standing with the feet comfortably forward, feet and legs together, spine and pelvis in a neutral position, arms by the side of the body.

Inhale to prepare.

Exhale to engage the abdominals, lengthen the spine and transfer the weight onto the right leg, ensure the pelvis remains level.

Inhale to bend the right knee over the 2nd metatarsal, ensure the pelvis remains stable and hip bones facing forwards.

Exhale to straighten the right knee.

Repeat the knee bends 10 times on the right side then 10 knee bends on the left side.

Technical Points

Try not to allow the pelvis to arch in the lumbar area and follow the ball, try to bend from the knees and keep the tailbone dropping directly to the floor.

Keep the arms relaxed by the sides of the body.

Keep the spine lengthened.

Keep the abdominals gently drawn back towards the spine.

Ensure the pelvis remains level, try not to hike one side of the pelvis up.

When bending the knees maintain the heels in contact with the floor.

Repetitions

10 Knee Bends Single Leg with the Ball.

Contra-indications

Avoid with knee pain or hip pain.

Basic Anatomy

Transversus Abdominus
Oblique Abdominals
Multifidus
Quadriceps
Erector Spinae
Gluteus Medius
Gluteus Maximus
Hip Flexors
Gastrocnemius
Soleus
Foot Flexors and Extensors

p-i-l-a-t-e-s
Core Stability Ball - Knee Bends - Level 2
Exercise 30 - Rise/Lower

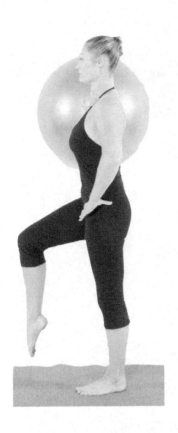

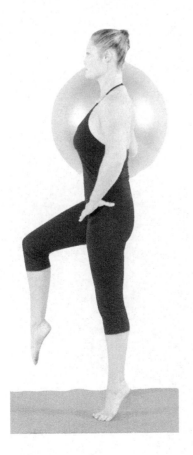

Exercise Focus

This exercise strengthens the calves, foot flexors and extensors.

Start Position

Standing side on to the wall, hold the ball between the body and the wall, standing with the feet comfortably hip width apart, spine and pelvis in a neutral position, arms by the side of the body. Raise the right leg to begin

Inhale to engage the abdominals and rise up onto the ball of the foot.

Exhale to lower the heel to the floor.

Inhale to rise up onto the balls of the feet, keep the ankles in line and weight distribution over the 2nd metatarsals.

Exhale to lower the heel to the floor with control.

Technical Points

Try not to allow the pelvis to arch in the lumbar area and follow the ball, try to bend from the knees and keep the tailbone dropping directly to the floor.

Keep the spine lengthened.

Keep the abdominals gently drawn back towards the spine.

When rising onto the balls of the feet, be aware of the ankles rolling outwards.

When bending the knees maintain the heels in contact with the floor.

Repetitions

10 Knee Bends with Rise/Lower with the Ball.

Contra-indications

Avoid with knee pain or hip pain.

Basic Anatomy

Transversus Abdominus
Oblique Abdominals
Multifidus
Quadriceps
Erector Spinae
Gluteus Medius
Gluteus Maximus
Hip Flexors
Gastrocnemius
Soleus
Foot Flexors and Extensors

p-i-l-a-t-e-s
Core Stability Ball - Lunges - Level 2
Exercise 31 - Twist

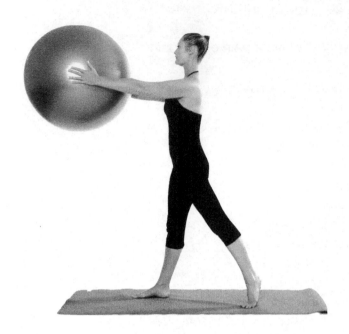

Exercise Focus

This exercise strengthens the abdominals, gluteals and quadriceps whilst challenging balance, core and pelvic stability.

Start Position

Standing on the mat, hold the ball in the hands, arms straight in front of the shoulders, place the right foot forward in line with the right hip joint, place the left foot behind the left hip, on the ball of the foot, pelvis in neutral, feet and legs parallel.

Inhale to engage the abdominals and bend both knees keeping most of the weight distribution on the right foot, maintain the arms in front of the body, simultaneously rotate the spine to the right taking the arms with the body, keep the arms directly in line with the shoulders.

Exhale to straighten the legs, maintain the arms at shoulder height and rotate the spine returning the body to the centre.

Repeat the exercise 10 Lunges Twist with the right leg in front, rotating to the right, then 10 with the left foot forward, rotating the spine to the left.

Technical Points

Keep the spine lengthened.

Try not to allow the pelvis to arch in the lumbar area and follow the ball, try to bend from the knees and keep the tailbone dropping directly to the floor.

Keep the abdominals gently drawn back towards the spine.

Try not to lean away from the side you are rotating to.

Ensure the pelvis remains level, try not to hike one side of the pelvis up.

Keep the arms in line with the shoulders when performing the exercise.

Repetitions

10 Lunges Twist with the Ball.

Contra-indications

Avoid with knee pain or hip pain.

Basic Anatomy

Transversus Abdominus
Oblique Abdominals
Multifidus
Erector Spinae
Quadriceps
Hamstrings
Gluteus Medius
Gluteus Maximus
Hip Flexors
Gastrocnemius
Soleus
Foot Flexors and Extensors

p-i-l-a-t-e-s
Core Stability Ball - Prone Leg Lifts - Level 1
Exercise 32 - Prone Single Leg Lifts

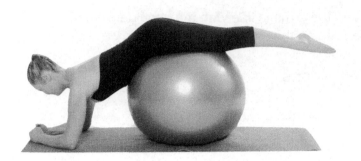

Exercise Focus

This exercise strengthens the hamstrings and gluteals whilst supporting the lumbar spine.

Start Position

Kneeling on the mat, place the body on the ball and walk the hands forward until the pelvis is on the ball, feet remain in contact with the mat, knees and feet hip width apart, legs straight, toes softly pointed, arms are bent at the elbows, hands slightly wider than shoulder width apart.

Inhale to engage the abdominals and adduct the legs.

Exhale to raise the right leg straight behind the hip, lift the right leg as high as possible without increasing the lumbar lordosis.

Inhale to keep the upper body still and lower the right leg to the mat.

Exhale to engage the abdominals and lift the left leg behind the hip, keep the left leg straight.

Inhale to lower the left leg to the mat with control.

Technical Points

Keep the spine lengthened.

Try not to collapse the shoulder blades together, keep the scapula still and isolate the press in and out from the arms only.

Keep the abdominals gently drawn back towards the spine.

Ensure the weight is evenly distributed on both arms.

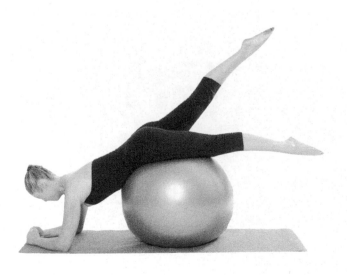

Keep the working leg straight on the lifting and lowering.

Try not to lift the working leg too high, do not change the curve in the lumbar spine or overuse the erector spinae muscles of the lumbar region.

Repetitions

5 Single Leg Lifts Prone each side on the Ball.

Contra-indications

Avoid with knee pain.

Avoid with neck pain.

Avoid with lower back pain.

Avoid with wrist pain.

Basic Anatomy

Transversus Abdominus
Oblique Abdominals
Multifidus
Erector Spinae
Middle and Lower Trapezius
Hamstrings
Gluteus Maximus

p-i-l-a-t-e-s
Core Stability Ball - Prone Leg Lifts - Level 2
Exercise 33 - Prone Double Leg Lifts

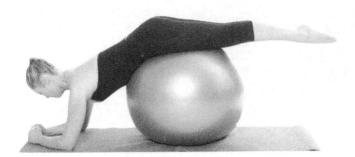

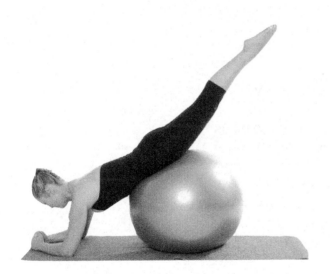

Exercise Focus

This exercise strengthens the hamstrings and gluteals whilst supporting the lumbar spine.

Start Position

Kneeling on the mat, place the body on the ball and walk the hands forward until the pelvis is on the ball, feet remain in contact with the mat, knees and feet adducted, toes softly pointed, arms are slightly bent at the elbows, hands slightly wider than shoulder width apart.

Inhale to engage the abdominals and adduct the legs.

Exhale to raise the legs straight behind the hips, lift the legs as high as possible without increasing the lumbar lordosis.

Inhale to keep the upper body still and lower the legs to the mat.

Exhale to engage the abdominals and lift both legs, keep the legs straight and together.

Inhale to lower the legs to the mat with control.

Technical Points

Keep the spine lengthened.

Try not to collapse the shoulder blades together, keep the scapula still and isolate the press in and out from the arms only.

Keep the abdominals gently drawn back towards the spine.

Ensure the weight is evenly distributed on both arms.

Keep the legs straight on the lifting and lowering.
Try not to lift the legs too high, do not change the
curve in the lumbar spine or overuse the erector
spinae muscles of the lumbar region.

Repetitions

6 Double Leg Lifts Prone on the Ball.

Contra-indications

Avoid with knee pain.

Avoid with neck pain.

Avoid with lower back pain.

Avoid with wrist pain.

Basic Anatomy

Transversus Abdominus
Oblique Abdominals
Multifidus
Erector Spinae
Middle and Lower Trapezius
Hamstrings
Gluteus Maximus

p-i-l-a-t-e-s
Core Stability Ball - Side Leg Series - Level 2
Exercise 34 - Lift/Lower

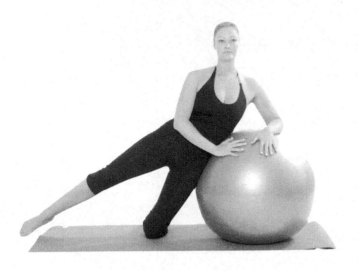

Exercise Focus

This exercise strengthens the hamstrings and the abductors of the hip.

Start Position

Place the ball on the left side of the body, lean the left hip onto the ball and place the left elbow on top of the ball, extend the right leg directly to the side, right foot pointed, place the right hand on the ball for stability, do not collapse into the shoulders.

Inhale to prepare and engage the abdominals.

Exhale to raise the right leg off the floor keeping the upper body still.

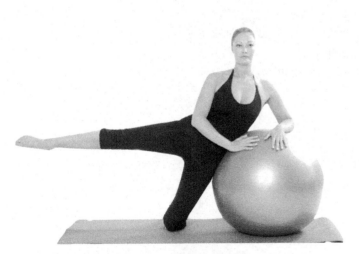
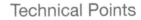

Inhale to lower the right foot to just off the floor, keep the right leg parallel.

Exhale to raise the right leg off the floor and continue the exercise.

Change sides and repeat the exercise.

Technical Points

Keep the body still on the ball as the leg lifts and lowers.

Maintain the scapula stability when resting the upper body on the ball.

Keep the pelvis still as the leg lifts and lowers, isolate the movement in the Gluteus Medius.

Repetitions

10 Side Leg Lifts on the Ball.

Contra-indications

Avoid with neck pain.

Avoid with lower back pain.

Avoid with shoulder pain or impingement pathology.

Basic Anatomy

Transversus Abdominus
Oblique Abdominals
Multifidus
Erector Spinae
Paraspinals
Quadratus Lumborum
Abductors of the Hip
Hamstrings

p-i-l-a-t-e-s
Core Stability Ball - Side Leg Series - Level 2
Exercise 35 - Circles

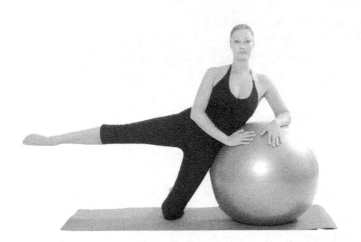

Exercise Focus

This exercise strengthens the hamstrings and abductors of the hip.

Start Position

Place the ball on the left side of the body, lean the left hip onto the ball and place the left elbow on top of the ball, extend the right leg directly to the side, right foot pointed, place the right hand on the ball for stability, do not collapse into the shoulders.

Inhale to prepare and engage the abdominals.

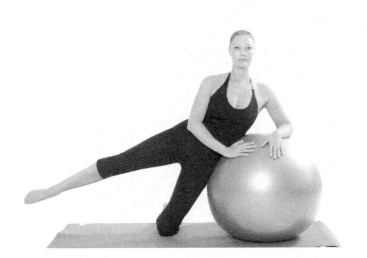

Exhale to raise the right leg off the floor keeping the upper body still.

Inhale to circle the right foot, 8 times clockwise, 8 times anti clockwise, inhaling for 2 small circles, exhaling for 2 small circles.

Inhale to lower the right foot to the floor.

Change sides and repeat the exercise.

Technical Points

Keep the body still on the ball as the leg lifts and lowers.

Maintain the scapula stability when resting the upper body on the ball.

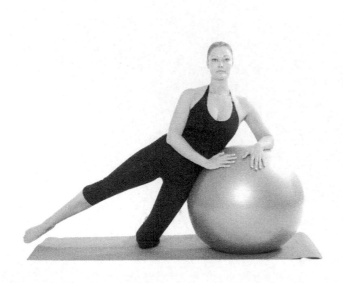

Keep the pelvis still as the leg lifts and lowers, isolate the movement in the hip abductors.

Repetitions

10 Side Leg Lifts with Circles on the Ball.

Contra-indications

Avoid with neck pain.

Avoid with lower back pain.

Avoid with shoulder pain or impingement pathology.

Basic Anatomy

Transversus Abdominus
Oblique Abdominals
Multifidus
Erector Spinae
Paraspinals
Quadratus Lumborum
Abductors of the Hip
Hamstrings

p-i-l-a-t-e-s
Core Stability Ball - Upper Back Lifts - Level 2
Exercise 36 - Hands Behind Head

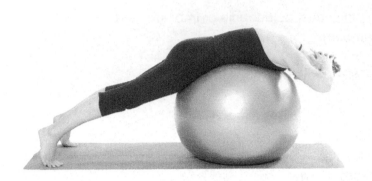

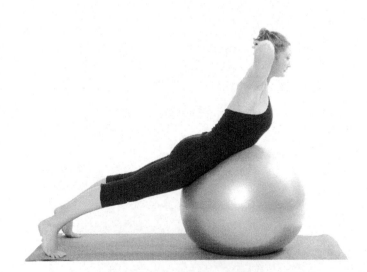

Exercise Focus

This exercise strengthens back extensors and gluteals.

Start Position

Kneeling on the mat, place the pelvis on the ball, feet are slightly wider than hip width apart, feet parallel, place the ball of the feet against the wall for support, fingers interlaced behind head, elbows to the sides of the body, ensure the body is in one straight line from the head to the feet.

Inhale to engage the abdominals and flex the upper spine forwards over the ball.

Exhale keeping the legs straight, lift the upper back and extend the spine as far back as comfortable.

Inhale to flex the upper spine forwards and continue the exercise.

Technical Points

Try to work from the mid thoracic muscle region of the back extensors, try not to over use the lumbar back extensors.

Keep the head in line with the spine.

Maintain the scapula stability.

Keep the legs straight and use the buttocks.

Repetitions

10 Upper Back Lifts each side on the Ball.

Contra-indications

Avoid with neck pain.

Avoid with lower back pain.

Avoid with wrist pain.

Basic Anatomy

Transversus Abdominus
Oblique Abdominals
Multifidus
Erector Spinae
Middle and Lower Trapezius
Hamstrings
Gluteus Maximus

p-i-l-a-t-e-s
Core Stability Ball - Full Back Stretch - Level 2
Exercise 37 - Back Stretch

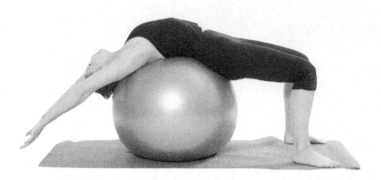

Exercise Focus

This exercise stretches the abdominals and hip flexors.

Start Position

Sitting on the ball, slowly roll the ball forwards to allow the spine to roll onto the ball, bend the knees and roll the spine over the ball until the head is resting, extend both arms over the ball behind the body and hold the position for 5 slow deep breaths.

Notice any sections of the spine that feel tight or stop the stretch if you feel uncomfortable, pain in the spine or dizziness.

Inhale to hold the position, then exhale to bring both arms forward and slowly press into the feet to roll the spine back up to a seated position.

Technical Points

Keep the spine lengthened.

Try not to allow the legs to roll inwards.

If there is shoulder pain keep the arms across the chest.

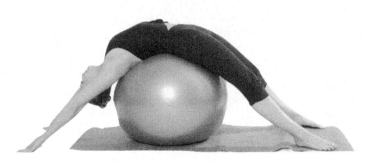

Repetitions

2 Full Back Stretches over the Ball.

Contra-indications

Avoid with lower back pain.

Avoid with neck pain or conditions such as whiplash injuries or osteoarthritis/osteoporosis.

Avoid with shoulder pain, dislocation pathology or shoulder impingement.

Basic Anatomy

Transversus Abdominus
Oblique Abdominals
Multifidus
Erector Spinae
Hamstrings
Illiopsoas
Paraspinals

p-i-l-a-t-e-s
Core Stability Ball - Pelvic Roll Up - Level 3
Exercise 38 - Hamstring Curl

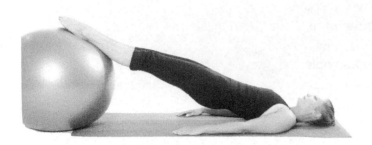

Exercise Focus

This exercise strengthens the hamstrings and gluteals whilst challenging neuromuscular control.

Start Position

Lying on the mat, place the legs on the ball, lower calves and heels on the ball, legs straight and adducted, arms rested by the sides of the body, feet softly pointed.

Inhale to prepare and engage the abdominals.

Exhale to curl the tailbone under and posteriorly tilt the pelvis (tuck the pelvis under) and curl the spine off the mat bone by bone, raise the pelvis off the floor.

Inhale to hold the position, relax the shoulders, keep the ball as still and stable as possible.

Exhale to bend the knees and roll the ball in towards the hips, controlling the movement from the hamstrings and abdominals.

Inhale to roll the ball in one straight line out extending both legs, keep the legs adducted and parallel.

Exhale to segmentally roll the spine back down onto the mat until the pelvis returns to a neutral spine.

Technical Points

Keep the shoulders, neck and arms relaxed.

Maintain the ball as still and stable as possible on the roll up and down through the spine.

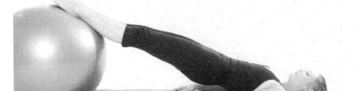

Keep the legs adducted and straight on the
and down through the spine.

Keep the legs parallel and adducted as the knees
bend in towards the chest, try not to drop the pelvis
towards the floor.

As the pelvis is lifted, try not to raise the pelvis too
high and arch the lower back.

Repetitions

5 Pelvic Roll Ups with Hamstring Curls on the Ball.

Contra-indications

Avoid with lower back pain or disc injuries.

Avoid with neck pain or whiplash pathology.

Avoid with knee pain or knee instability.

Avoid during pregnancy.

Basic Anatomy

Transversus Abdominus
Oblique Abdominals
Rectus Abdominus
Multifidus
Hamstrings
Gluteus Maximus
Gluteus Medius
Quadriceps
Illiopsoas
Deep Neck Flexors
Scapula Stabilisers

p-i-l-a-t-e-s
Core Stability Ball - Walk Downs - Level 3
Exercise 39 - Arm Circles

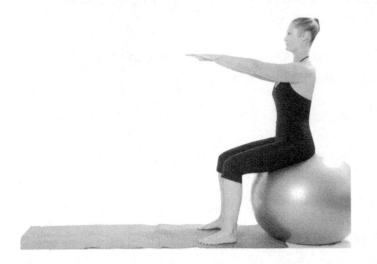

Exercise Focus

This exercise mobilises the spine and strengthens the abdominals whilst stretching the pectorals and anterior aspect of the shoulder joint.

Start Position

Sitting on the ball, feet and knees hip width apart, arms raised forward at shoulder height, scapula stabilised, pelvis and spine in a neutral position.

Inhale to prepare and engage the abdominals.

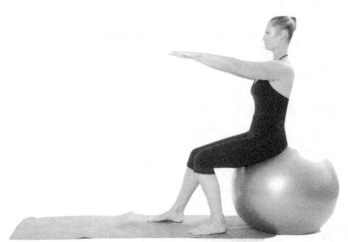

Exhale to curl the tailbone under and roll the spine down onto the ball with control whilst simultaneously walking the feet forwards, walk the feet forwards until your head, neck and shoulders are comfortably placed onto the ball, arms will be directly above the shoulders.

Inhale to hold the position, keep lifting the pelvis and engage the buttocks.

Exhale to circle the arms behind the head and to the sides of the body.

Inhale to continue to circle the arms down to the hips and up towards the ceiling.

Repeat the circles 3 times, then,

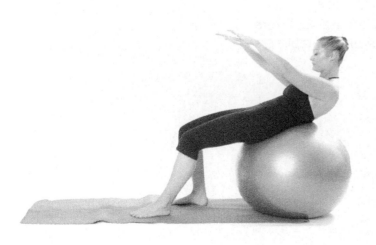

Exhale to engage the abdominals and press through the feet whilst simultaneously drawing the chin towards the chest and roll the spine back up to a sitting position.   Technical Points

Keep the rolling action down and up off the ball smooth and controlled.

Use a non slip mat on the floor if necessary.

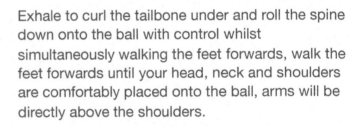

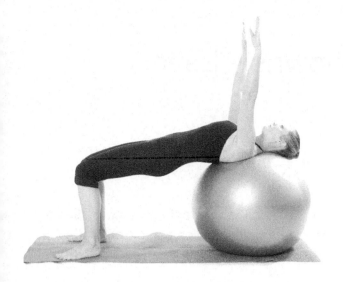

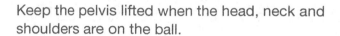

Keep the pelvis lifted when the head, neck and shoulders are on the ball.

Maintain the scapula stability at all times.

Repetitions

5 Walk Downs with 3 Arm Circles on the Ball.

Contra-indications

Avoid with lower back pain or disc injuries.

Avoid with neck pain or whiplash pathology.

Avoid with shoulder injuries or pathology such as shoulder dislocation or sublaxations.

Avoid during pregnancy.

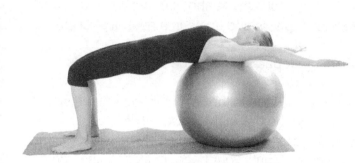

Basic Anatomy

Transversus Abdominus
Oblique Abdominals
Rectus Abdominus
Multifidus
Hamstrings
Quadriceps
Illiopsoas
Deep Neck Flexors
Scapula Stabilisers

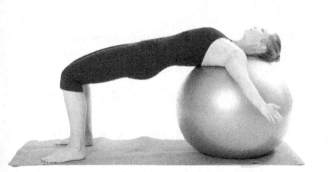

p-i-l-a-t-e-s
Core Stability Ball - Walk Downs - Level 3
Exercise 40 - Knee Lifts

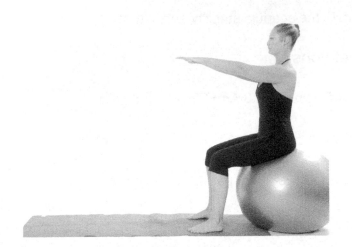

Exercise Focus

This exercise mobilises the spine and strengthens the abdominals whilst challenging co-ordination and control.

Start Position

Sitting on the ball, feet and knees hip width apart, arms raised forward at shoulder height, scapula stabilised, pelvis and spine in a neutral position.

Inhale to prepare and engage the abdominals.

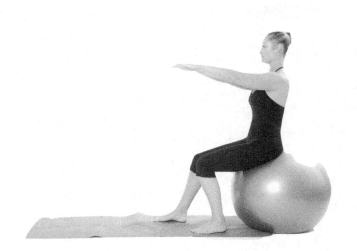

Exhale to curl the tailbone under and roll the spine down onto the ball with control whilst simultaneously walking the feet forwards, walk the feet forwards until your head, neck and shoulders are comfortably placed onto the ball, arms will be directly above the shoulders.

Inhale to hold the position, keep lifting the pelvis and engage the buttocks.

Exhale to lift the right foot off the ground with control.

Inhale to lower the right foot to the floor.

Exhale to lift the left foot off the floor keeping the pelvis steady and stable.

Inhale to lower the left foot to the floor with control.

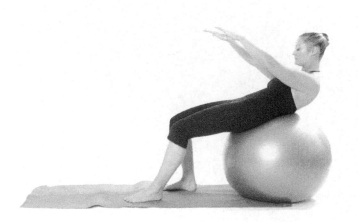

Exhale to engage the abdominals and press through the feet whilst simultaneously drawing the chin towards the chest and roll the spine back up to a sitting position.

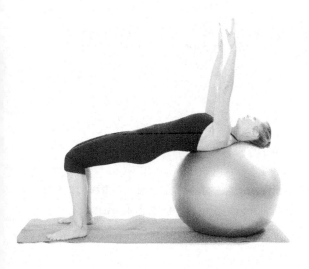

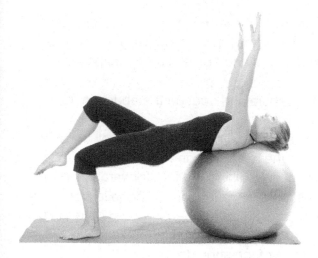

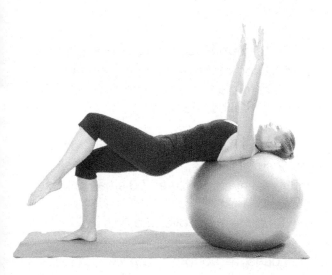

Technical Points

Keep the rolling action down and up off the ball smooth and controlled.

Use a non slip mat on the floor if necessary.

Keep the pelvis lifted when the head, neck and shoulders are on the ball.

Maintain the scapula stability at all times.

Repetitions

3 Walk Downs with 3 Knee Lifts on each side on the Ball.

Contra-indications

Avoid with lower back pain or disc injuries.

Avoid with neck pain or whiplash pathology.

Avoid during pregnancy.

Basic Anatomy

Transversus Abdominus
Oblique Abdominals
Rectus Abdominus
Multifidus
Hamstrings
Gluteus Maximus
Gluteus Medius
Quadriceps
Illiopsoas
Deep Neck Flexors
Scapula Stabilisers

p-i-l-a-t-e-s
Core Stability Ball - Abdominal Curls - Level 3
Exercise 41 - Pulses

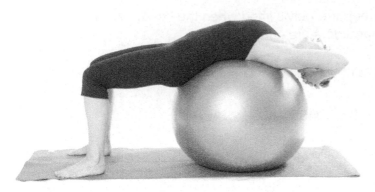

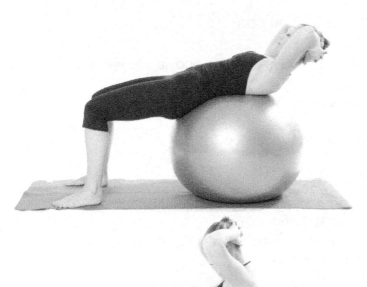

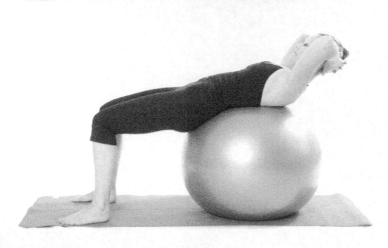

Exercise Focus

This exercise mobilises the spine and strengthens the upper obliques and rectus abdominus.

Start Position

Sitting on the ball, feet and knees hip width apart, arms raised forward at shoulder height, scapula stabilised, pelvis and spine in a neutral position.

Inhale to prepare and engage the abdominals.

Exhale to curl the tailbone under and roll the spine down onto the ball with control whilst simultaneously walking the feet forwards, walk the feet forwards until your head, tailbone is just off the ball, shoulders are comfortably placed onto the ball, interlace the hands behind the head and elbows open in front of the shoulders.

Inhale to extend the spine over the ball as far back as comfortable.

Exhale to curl the upper spine forwards starting from the small nod of the head, curl the head, neck, shoulders forward maintaining a stable pelvis, try not to curl the tailbone under.

Pulse the shoulders and upper body forwards, inhaling for 2 small pulses, exhaling for 2 small pulses until you have completed 20 small pulses.

Inhale to extend the spine over the ball.

Exhale to engage the abdominals and press through the feet whilst simultaneously drawing the chin towards the chest and roll the spine back up to a sitting position.

Technical Points

Keep the pulses small and controlled, working from the abdominals.

Try not to pull on the neck with the hands.

Keep the rolling action down and up off the ball smooth and controlled.

Keep the elbows forwards in the peripheral vision when curling and extending the spine.

Keep the eye focus on the abdominals when curling forward, try not to extend the neck and look up to the ceiling.

Try not to arch the lumbar spine when curling back over the ball.

Use a non slip mat on the floor if necessary.

Maintain the scapula stability at all times.

Repetitions

10 Abdominal Pulses Forward on the Ball.

Contra-indications

Avoid with lower back pain or disc injuries.

Avoid with neck pain or whiplash pathology.

Avoid during pregnancy.

Basic Anatomy

Transversus Abdominus
Oblique Abdominals
Rectus Abdominus
Multifidus
Hamstrings
Quadriceps
Illiopsoas
Deep Neck Flexors
Scapula Stabilisers

p-i-l-a-t-e-s
Core Stability Ball - Abdominal Curls - Level 3
Exercise 42 - Around The World

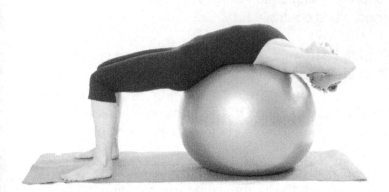

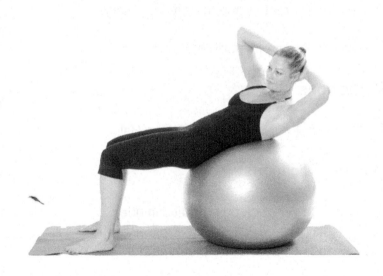

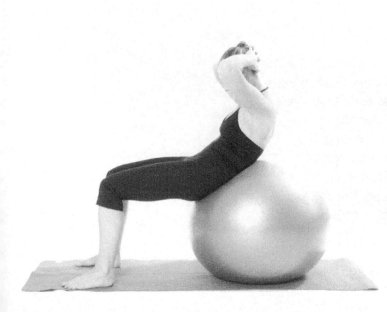

Exercise Focus

This exercise mobilises the thoracic spine and strengthens the abdominals.

Start Position

Sitting on the ball, feet and knees hip width apart, arms raised forward at shoulder height, scapula stabilised, pelvis and spine in a neutral position.

Inhale to prepare and engage the abdominals.

Exhale to curl the tailbone under and roll the spine down onto the ball with control whilst simultaneously walking the feet forwards, walk the feet forwards until your head, tailbone is just off the ball, shoulders are comfortably placed onto the ball, interlace the hands behind the head and elbows open in front of the shoulders.

Inhale to extend the spine over the ball as far back as comfortable.

Exhale to curl the upper spine forwards starting from the small nod of the head, curl the head, neck, shoulders forward maintaining a stable pelvis, try not to curl the tailbone under, curl the upper body to the right side.

Inhale and maintain the curl up, bring the shoulders to the centre.

Exhale to maintain the curl up and rotate the shoulders and spine to the left shoulder blade.

Inhale to extend the spine over the ball.

Repeat the exercise 4 times curling to the right, then 4 times curling towards the left, then,

Exhale to engage the abdominals and press through the feet whilst simultaneously drawing the chin towards the chest and roll the spine back up to a sitting position.

Technical Points

Try not to pull on the neck with the hands, maintain the shoulders relaxed.

Keep the rolling action down and up off the ball smooth and controlled.

Keep the elbows forwards in the peripheral vision when curling and extending the spine.

Keep the eye focus on the abdominals when curling forward, try not to extend the neck and look up to the ceiling.

Try not to arch the lumbar spine when curling back over the ball.

Maintain the scapula stability at all times.

Repetitions

4 Around the World each direction on the Ball.

Contra-indications

Avoid with lower back pain or disc injuries.

Avoid with neck pain or whiplash pathology.

Avoid during pregnancy.

Basic Anatomy

Transversus Abdominus
Oblique Abdominals
Rectus Abdominus
Multifidus
Hamstrings
Quadriceps
Illiopsoas
Deep Neck Flexors
Scapula Stabilisers

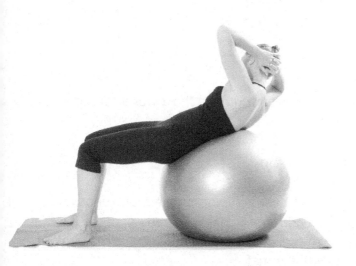

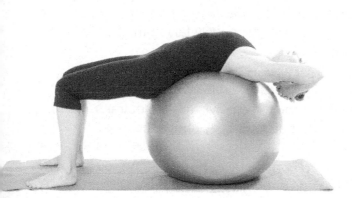

p-i-l-a-t-e-s
Core Stability Ball - Small Pelvic Lifts - Level 3
Exercise 43 - Lower Abdominals

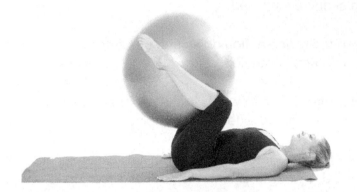

Exercise Focus

This exercise strengthens the lower abdominals and hip flexors.

Start Position

Lying on the semi-supine on the mat, knees and feet hip width apart, pelvis in neutral, place the ball between the knees and inner thighs, arms straight, alongside the mat.

Inhale to prepare and engage the abdominals.

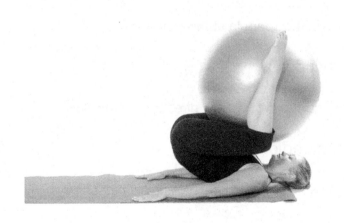

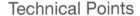

Exhale to initiate the tailbone curling under and posteriorly tilt the pelvis and curl the pelvis off the mat whilst simultaneously taking the ball towards the chest.

Inhale to control the roll down of the pelvis and spine returning the pelvis to the neutral position, return the ball to directly above the hips.

Exhale to curl the tailbone under and roll the pelvis off the mat and repeat the exercise.

Technical Points

Keep the arms and shoulders relaxed as much as possible.

Maintain a slight squeeze with the adductors.

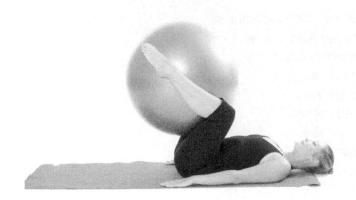

Keep the head still on the roll over and return, be aware of the chin lifting.

Repetitions

8 Small Pelvic Lifts with the Ball.

Contra-indications

Avoid with lower back pain or disc injuries.

Avoid with neck pain or pathology such as whiplash or osteoarthritis.

Avoid during pregnancy.

Basic Anatomy

Transversus Abdominus
Oblique Abdominals
Rectus Abdominus
Multifidus
Hip Flexors
Illiopsoas
Hamstrings
Adductors
Scapula Stabilisers
Arm Extensors

p-i-l-a-t-e-s
Core Stability Ball - The One Hundred - Level 3
Exercise 44 - Feet On Ball

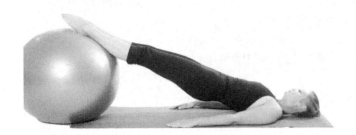

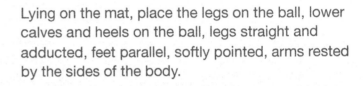

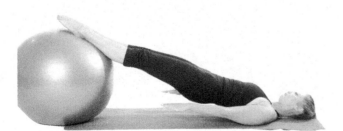

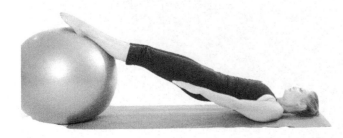

Exercise Focus

This exercise builds stamina in the gluteals, abdominals and hamstrings whilst challenging breathing and co-ordination.

Start Position

Lying on the mat, place the legs on the ball, lower calves and heels on the ball, legs straight and adducted, feet parallel, softly pointed, arms rested by the sides of the body.

Inhale to prepare and engage the abdominals.

Exhale to curl the tailbone under and posteriorly tilt the pelvis (tuck the pelvis under) and curl the spine off the mat bone by bone, raise the pelvis off the floor.

Inhale to hold the position, keep the ball as still and stable as possible, raise the arms slightly off the mat maintaining the scapula stability.

Exhale for a count of 5 small beats with the arms, inhale for 5 small beats of the arms.

When you have completed 10 sets of inhaling for 5 beats and exhaling for 5 beats.

Inhale to hold the pelvis lifted, lower the arms to the mat.

Exhale to segmentally roll the spine back down onto the mat until the pelvis returns to a neutral spine.

Technical Points

Keep the shoulders open and the scapula stabilised.

Maintain the ball as still and stable as possible as the arms are beating at the sides of the body.

Keep the legs adducted and straight.

As the pelvis is lifted, try not to raise the pelvis too high and arch the lower back.

Keep the neck relaxed.

Repetitions

1 Set of The One Hundred on the Ball.

Contra-indications

Avoid with lower back pain or disc injuries.

Avoid with neck pain or whiplash pathology.

Avoid during pregnancy.

Basic Anatomy

Transversus Abdominus
Oblique Abdominals
Rectus Abdominus
Multifidus
Hamstrings
Quadriceps
Illiopsoas
Deep Neck Flexors
Scapula Stabilisers

p-i-l-a-t-e-s
Core Stability Ball - Single Leg Stretch - Level 3
Exercise 45 - Hands Up

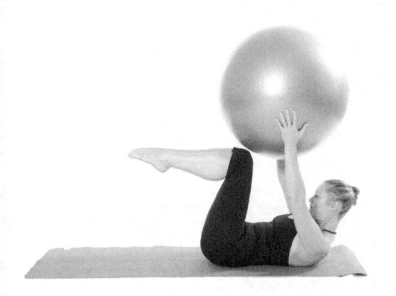

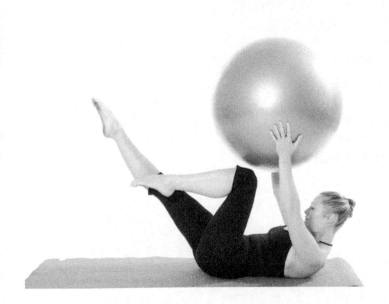

Exercise Focus

This exercise strengthens the abdominals, hip flexors and scapula stabilisers.

Start Position

Lying on the semi-supine on the mat, knees and feet hip width apart, pelvis in neutral, place the ball in the hands, arms straight, directly above the shoulders, stabilise the scapula.

Inhale to prepare and engage the abdominals.

Exhale to curl the upper spine forward, draw the chin gently towards the chest, curl the head, neck and shoulders off the mat simultaneously lowering the ball forwards, bring the right leg up to the "table top" position, then the left.

Inhale to hold the position.

Exhale to extend the right leg out to 45° maintain the curl up of the upper spine.

Inhale to simultaneously bring the right leg in towards the chest, return the right leg to the "table top" position whilst simultaneously extending the left leg away from the hip out to 45°.

Exhale to simultaneously bring the left leg in towards the chest, return the left leg to the "table top" position and repeat the exercise.

Technical Points

Maintain the pelvis and spine in neutral as the leg fully extends away from the hip, try not to allow the lumbar lordosis to increase.

Keep the shoulder blades drawing down the back.

Maintain the eye focus on the abdominals to keep the head on top of the spine.

Keep the navel drawn gently back towards the spine throughout the entire exercise.

Keep both legs parallel.

Try not to posteriorly tilt the pelvis under as the leg draws in towards the body.

Repetitions

10 Single Leg Stretch Hands Up on the Ball.

Contra-indications

Avoid with lower back pain or disc injuries.

Avoid with neck pain or pathology such as whiplash or osteoarthritis.

Avoid during pregnancy.

Basic Anatomy

Transversus Abdominus
Oblique Abdominals
Rectus Abdominus
Multifidus
Quadriceps
Hip Flexors
Illiopsoas
Scapula Stabilisers
Arm Extensors

p-i-l-a-t-e-s
Core Stability Ball - Upper Back Lifts - Level 3
Exercise 46 - Arms Forward

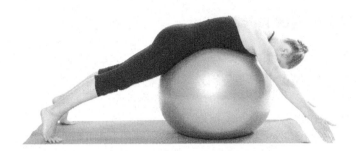

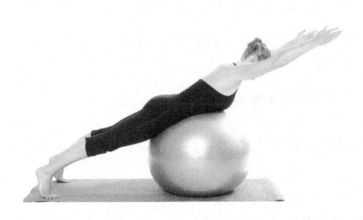

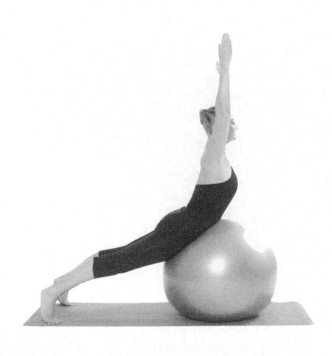

Exercise Focus

This exercise strengthens the spinal extensors with an increased load.

Start Position

Kneeling on the mat, place the pelvis on the ball, feet are slightly wider than hip width apart, feet parallel, place the ball of the feet against the wall for support, arms reaching over head, scapula stabilised, ensure the body is in one straight line from the head to the feet.

Inhale to engage the abdominals and flex the upper spine forwards over the ball.

Exhale keeping the legs straight, lift the upper back and extend the spine as far back as comfortable, keep the arms straight and in line with the shoulders.

Inhale to flex the upper spine forwards and continue the exercise.

Technical Points

Try to work from the mid thoracic muscle region of the back extensors, try not to over use the lumbar back extensors.

Keep the head in line with the spine.

Maintain the scapula stability.

Keep the legs straight and use the buttocks.

Repetitions

10 Upper Back Lifts with Straight Arms each side on the Ball.

Contra-indications

Avoid with neck pain.

Avoid with lower back pain.

Basic Anatomy

Transversus Abdominus
Oblique Abdominals
Multifidus
Erector Spinae
Middle and Lower Trapezius
Hamstrings
Gluteus Maximus
Arm Extensors

p-i-l-a-t-e-s
Core Stability Ball - Side Lifts - Level 3
Exercise 47 - Side Lift

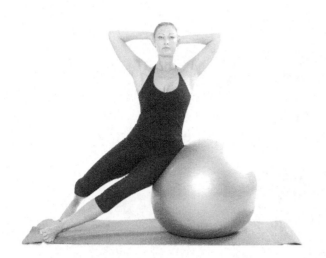

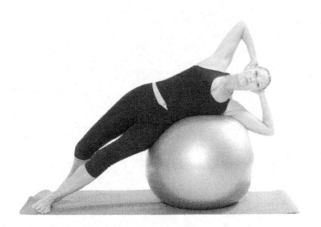

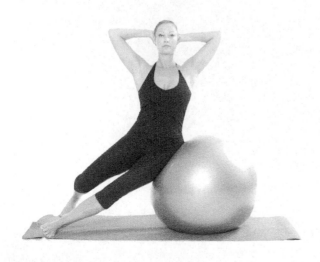

Exercise Focus

This exercise strengthens and stretches the side flexors of the spine and torso.

Start Position

Kneeling on the mat, place the ball on the left side of the body, place the hip left hip on the ball, feet are slightly wider than hip width apart, left foot in front, right foot on the ball of the foot, hands interlaced behind the head, scapula stabilised, ensure the body is in one straight line from the head to the hip.

Inhale to engage the abdominals and side flex the upper spine forwards over the ball to the left.

Exhale to side flex the spine towards the right hip, keep the scapula stabilised.

Inhale to side flex the spine to the left and continue the exercise.

Technical Points

Keep the ball stable throughout the exercise.

Keep the movement flowing.

Try not to rotate the shoulders forwards on the side flexion.

Keep the pelvis stable, try not to rotate the pelvis backwards to over use the oblique abdominals, keep the movement pure side flexion.

Repetitions

10 Side Lifts on the Ball.

Contra-indications

Avoid with neck pain.

Avoid with lower back pain.

Avoid with shoulder pain or impingement pathology.

Basic Anatomy

Transversus Abdominus
Oblique Abdominals
Multifidus
Erector Spinae
Paraspinals
Quadratus Lumborum
Middle and Lower Trapezius
Hamstrings
Adductors
Gluteus Maximus
Arm Extensors

p-i-l-a-t-e-s
Core Stability Ball - Side Lying Lifts - Level 3
Exercise 48 - Ball Lifts

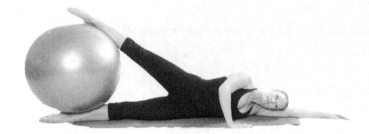

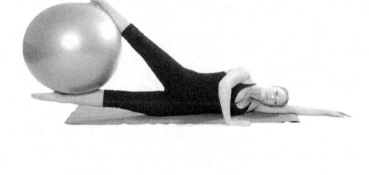

Exercise Focus

This exercise strengthens the adductors and side flexors of the spine and torso.

Start Position

Lying on the left side of the body on the mat, place the ball between the ankles, legs straight, feet parallel, right hand placed on the mat in front of the right shoulder.

Inhale to prepare and engage the abdominals.

Exhale to squeeze the ball, raise both legs off the mat, keep the body still and stable.

Inhale to lower the legs to the mat with control.

Exhale to lift both legs off the mat, keep the head rested on the left arm.

Inhale to lower the legs with control and continue the exercise.

Change sides and repeat the exercise.

Technical Points

Keep the legs straight and parallel.

Keep the pelvis stable, try not to rotate the pelvis backwards to over use the oblique abdominals, keep the movement pure side flexion.

Keep a gentle squeeze on the ball throughout the exercise.

Try not to place too much pressure on the front hand.

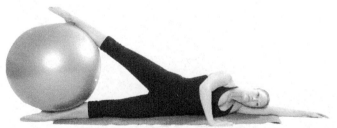

Repetitions

10 Lying Side Lifts on the Ball.

Contra-indications

Avoid with neck pain.

Avoid with lower back pain.

Avoid with shoulder pain or impingement pathology.

Basic Anatomy

Transversus Abdominus
Oblique Abdominals
Multifidus
Erector Spinae
Paraspinals
Quadratus Lumborum
Adductors

p-i-l-a-t-e-s
Core Stability Ball - Side Lying Lifts - Level 3
Exercise 49 - Rotation

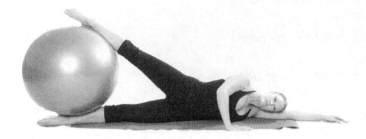

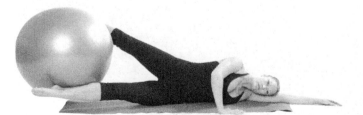

Exercise Focus

This exercise strengthens the adductors and side flexors of the spine and torso.

Start Position

Lying on the left side of the body on the mat, place the ball between the ankles, legs straight, feet parallel, right hand placed on the mat in front of the right shoulder.

Inhale to prepare and engage the abdominals.

Exhale to squeeze the ball, raise both legs off the mat, keep the body still and stable.

Inhale to hold the legs lifted and rotate the right leg forward, keep the pelvis stable.

Exhale to rotate the right leg backwards whilst simultaneously the left leg rotates forwards.

Inhale to rotate the right leg forwards whilst simultaneously rotate the left leg backwards and continue the exercise.

Change sides and repeat the exercise.

Technical Points

Keep the legs straight.

Keep the pelvis stable, try not to rotate the pelvis backwards to over use the oblique abdominals, keep the movement pure side flexion.

Keep a gentle squeeze on the ball throughout the exercise.

Try not to place too much pressure on the front hand.

Repetitions

10 Lying Side Lifts with Rotation on the Ball.

Contra-indications

Avoid with neck pain.

Avoid with lower back pain.

Avoid with shoulder pain or impingement pathology.

Basic Anatomy

Transversus Abdominus
Oblique Abdominals
Multifidus
Erector Spinae
Paraspinals
Quadratus Lumborum
Adductors

p-i-l-a-t-e-s
Core Stability Ball - Side Lying Lifts - Level 3
Exercise 50 - Adductor Squeezes

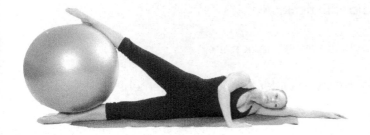

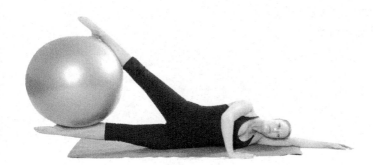

Exercise Focus

This exercise strengthens the hip adductors and side flexors of the spine and torso.

Start Position

Lying on the left side of the body on the mat, place the ball between the ankles, legs straight, feet pointed, right hand placed on the mat in front of the right shoulder.

Inhale to prepare and engage the abdominals to squeeze the ball, raise both legs off the mat, keep the body still and stable.

Exhale to hold the position and gently squeeze the ball 10 times keeping the spine and pelvis as stable as possible.

Inhale to lower the legs with control and continue the exercise.

Change sides and repeat the exercise.

Technical Points

Keep the legs straight and parallel.

Keep the pelvis stable, try not to rotate the pelvis backwards to over use the oblique abdominals, keep the movement pure side flexion.

Keep a gentle squeeze on the ball throughout the exercise.

Try not to place too much pressure on the front hand.

Repetitions

10 Lying Side Lifts with Adductor Squeezes on the Ball.

Contra-indications

Avoid with neck pain.

Avoid with lower back pain.

Avoid with shoulder pain or impingement pathology.

Basic Anatomy

Transversus Abdominus
Oblique Abdominals
Multifidus
Erector Spinae
Paraspinals
Quadratus Lumborum
Adductors

p-i-l-a-t-e-s
Core Stability Ball - Side Leg Series - Level 3
Exercise 51 - Forward/Back

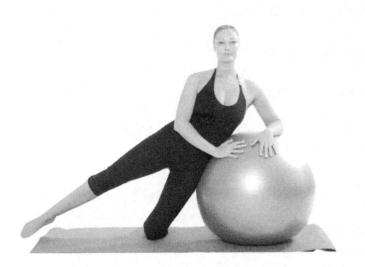

Exercise Focus

This exercise strengthens the hamstrings and abductors of the hip whilst challenging pelvic stability.

Start Position

Place the ball on the left side of the body, lean the left hip onto the ball and place the left elbow on top of the ball, extend the right leg directly to the side, right foot pointed, place the right hand on the ball for stability, do not collapse into the shoulders.

Inhale to prepare and engage the abdominals.

Exhale to raise the right leg off the floor keeping the upper body still.

Inhale to sweep the right leg forward of the hip, keep the pelvis stable.

Exhale to sweep the right leg behind the hip without losing the neutral pelvis.

Inhale to sweep the right leg forward of the hip and continue the exercise.

Change sides and repeat the exercise.

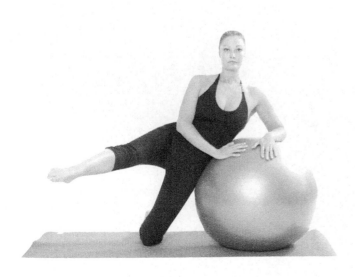

Technical Points

Keep the body still on the ball as the leg sweeps forward and back.

Maintain the scapula stability when resting the upper body on the ball.

Keep the pelvis still as the leg lifts and lowers, isolate the movement in the hip abductors.

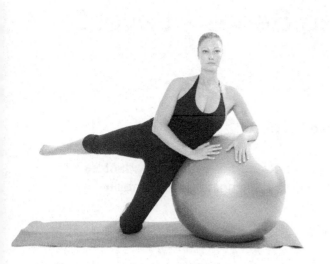

Repetitions

10 Side Leg Lifts Forward/Back on the Ball.

Contra-indications

Avoid with neck pain.

Avoid with lower back pain.

Avoid with shoulder pain or impingement pathology.

Basic Anatomy

Transversus Abdominus
Oblique Abdominals
Multifidus
Erector Spinae
Paraspinals
Quadratus Lumborum
Abductors of the Hip
Hamstrings

p-i-l-a-t-e-s
Core Stability Ball - Side Leg Series - Level 3
Exercise 52 - Pulses Up

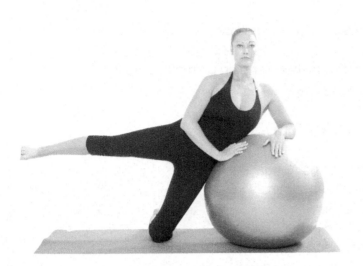

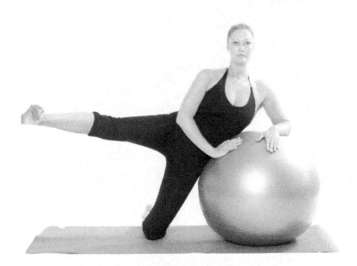

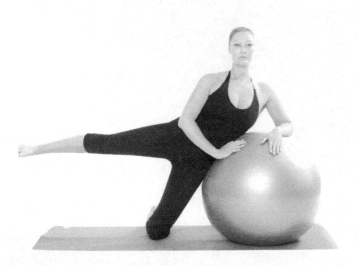

Exercise Focus

This exercise strengthens the hip abductors and gluteals whilst challenging pelvic stability.

Start Position

Place the ball on the left side of the body, lean the left hip onto the ball and place the left elbow on top of the ball, extend the right leg directly to the side, right foot flexed, place the right hand on the ball for stability, do not collapse into the shoulders.

Inhale to prepare and engage the abdominals.

Exhale to raise the right leg off the floor keeping the upper body still, flex the right foot.

Inhale to pulse the right leg upwards for 10 small pulses, inhaling for 2 pulses and exhaling for 2 small pulses.

Inhale to lower the right leg with control and continue the exercise.

Change sides and repeat the exercise.

To add a challenge when raising the leg control the leg forwards 45 degrees and pulse the leg up 10 times.

Technical Points

Keep the body still on the ball as the working leg pulses upwards.

Maintain the scapula stability when resting the upper body on the ball.

Keep the pelvis still as the leg lifts and lowers, try not to bounce the movement into the waistline.

Try not to rotate the pelvis forwards

Repetitions

10 Side Leg Lifts Small Pulses Up on the Ball.

Contra-indications

Avoid with neck pain.

Avoid with lower back pain.

Avoid with shoulder pain or impingement pathology.

Basic Anatomy

Transversus Abdominus
Oblique Abdominals
Multifidus
Erector Spinae
Paraspinals
Quadratus Lumborum
Abductors of the Hip
Hamstrings

-i-l-a-t-e-s
Core Stability Ball - Knee Stretches - Level 3
Exercise 53 - On Elbow

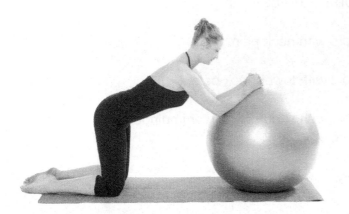

Exercise Focus

This exercise strengthens the abdominals, scapula stabilisers and challenges core stability.

Start Position

Kneeling on the mat, feet and knees hip width apart, place the ball in front of the body, place the elbows and forearms resting on the top of the ball, spine and pelvis in neutral, stabilise the shoulders down the back, keep the head in line with the spine.

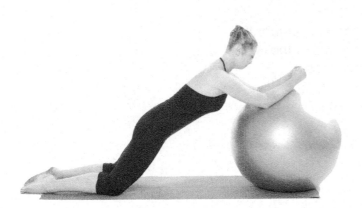

Inhale to engage the abdominals and slowly roll the body and the ball simultaneously away from the hips.

Exhale to maintain the neutral pelvis and spine and slowly roll the ball in towards the hips, keep the scapula stabilised.

Inhale to maintain the abdominals drawn back towards the spine and slowly roll the ball forwards as far as comfortable and repeat the exercise.

Technical Points

Try not to arch the lower back as the ball rolls forwards and backwards, maintain a neutral spine.

Keep control of the ball in both directions.

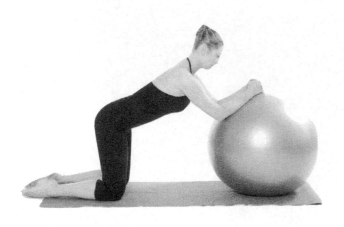

Try not to collapse the upper thoracic spine and bring the scapula together.

Keep the shoulders drawn down the back and head in line with the spine.

Repetitions

10 Knee Stretches on the Ball.

Contra-indications

Avoid with neck pain.

Avoid with lower back pain.

Avoid with shoulder pain or impingement
pathology.

Basic Anatomy

Transversus Abdominus
Oblique Abdominals
Multifidus
Erector Spinae
Hip Flexors
Quadriceps
Hamstrings
Serratus Anterior
Rhomboids
Latissimus Dorsi
Middle and Lower Trapezius
Pectorals

p-i-l-a-t-e-s
Stability Ball - Pelvic Roll Up - Level 4
Exercise 54 - Leg Lift

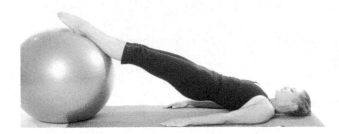

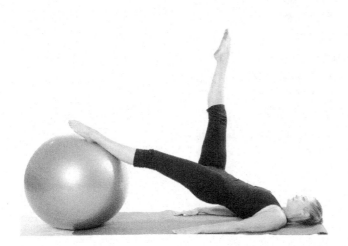

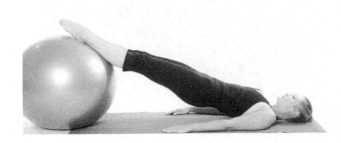

Exercise Focus

This exercise strengthens the hamstrings and gluteals whilst challenging pelvic and core stability.

Start Position

Lying on the mat, place the legs on the ball, lower calves and heels on the ball, legs straight and adducted, arms rested by the sides of the body, feet softly pointed.

Inhale to prepare and engage the abdominals.

Exhale to curl the tailbone under and posteriorly tilt the pelvis (tuck the pelvis under) and curl the spine off the mat bone by bone, raise the pelvis off the floor.

Inhale to hold the position, relax the shoulders, keep the ball as still and stable as possible.

Exhale to engage the right buttock and maintain a stable pelvis as you lift the left leg just off the ball.

Inhale to lower the left leg back to the ball.

Exhale to engage the left buttock and raise the right foot slightly off the ball.

Inhale to lower the right foot back to the ball.

Exhale to segmentally roll the spine back down onto the mat until the pelvis returns to a neutral spine.

Exercise Progression

If you are able to roll up and down the spine with the ball still and stable, try raising both arms slightly off the mat to further challenge core stability.

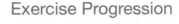

Technical Points

Keep the shoulders, neck and arms relaxed.

Maintain the ball as still and stable as possible.

Keep the legs adducted and straight.

As the pelvis is lifted, try not to raise the pelvis too high and arch the lower back.

Repetitions

2 Pelvic Roll Ups with 2 Leg Lifts each side on the Ball.

Contra-indications

Avoid with lower back pain or disc injuries.

Avoid with neck pain or whiplash pathology.

Avoid during pregnancy.

Basic Anatomy

Transversus Abdominus
Oblique Abdominals
Rectus Abdominus
Multifidus
Hamstrings
Gluteus Medius
Gluteus Maximus
Quadriceps
Illiopsoas
Deep Neck Flexors
Scapula Stabilisers

p-i-l-a-t-e-s
Stability Ball - Abdominal Curls - Level 4
Exercise 55 - Knee Lift

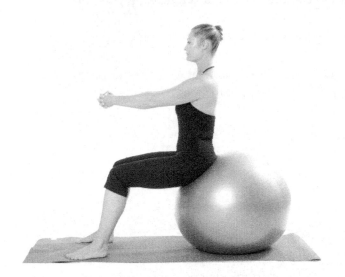

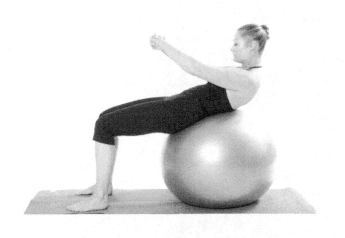

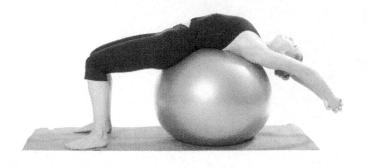

Exercise Focus

This exercise challenges balance, control, co-ordination and flowing movements whilst strengthening the hip flexors and abdominals, it also challenges pelvic stability.

Start Position

Sitting on the ball, feet and knees hip width apart, arms raised forward at shoulder height, scapula stabilised, pelvis and spine in a neutral position.

Inhale to prepare and engage the abdominals.

Exhale to curl the tailbone under and roll the spine down onto the ball with control whilst simultaneously walking the feet forwards, walk the feet forwards until you are half way down on the ball, the pelvis and sacrum are on the ball, clasp one hand in the other, arms straight and in front of the body.

Inhale to roll the upper body over the ball, extend the spine over the ball as far back as comfortable whilst simultaneously taking the arms behind the head.

Exhale to raise the arms forward whilst simultaneously curling the upper spine forwards starting from the small nod of the head, curl the head, neck, shoulders forward maintaining a stable pelvis, try not to curl the tailbone under, as you curl the body forwards simultaneously raise the right foot off the mat.

Inhale to lower the right foot to the mat whilst simultaneously rolling the spine backwards, extend the spine over the ball and take both arms behind the head.

Repeat the exercise 3 times each side, alternating the leg lifted, then,

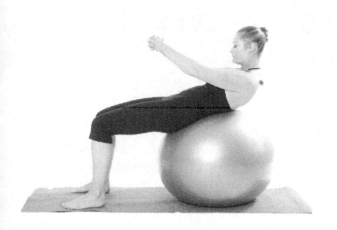

Exhale to engage the abdominals and press through the feet whilst simultaneously drawing the chin towards the chest and roll the spine back up to a sitting position.

Technical Points

Keep the movement forwards and backwards controlled and flowing.

Keep the eye focus on the abdominals when curling forward, try not to extend the neck and look up to the ceiling.

Try not to arch the lumbar spine when curling back over the ball.

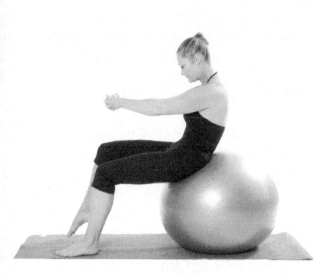

Maintain the scapula stability at all times, keeping the shoulders down particularly as the spine curls forwards.

Try not to press into the thoracic area and protract the shoulder blades.

Repetitions

3 Abdominal Curls with Knee Lifts on each side on the Ball.

Contra-indications

Avoid with lower back pain or disc injuries.

Avoid with neck pain or whiplash pathology.

Avoid during pregnancy.

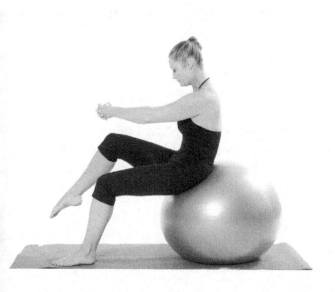

Basic Anatomy

Transversus Abdominus
Rectus Abdominus
Hamstrings
Gluteus Medius
Quadriceps
Illiopsoas
Hip Flexors
Deep Neck Flexors
Scapula Stabilisers

p-i-l-a-t-e-s
Stability Ball - The One Hundred - Level 4
Exercise 56 - Ball Between Ankles

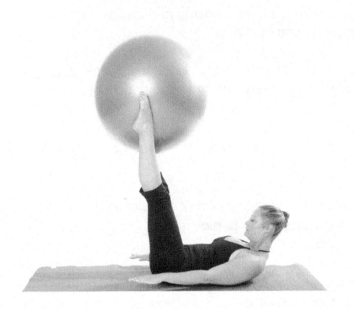

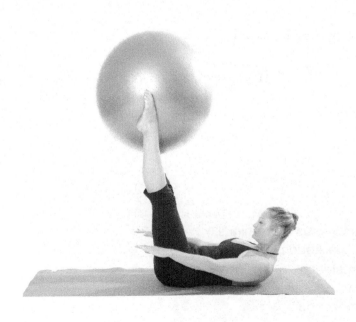

Exercise Focus

This exercise builds stamina in the abdominals and adductors whilst challenging breathing and co-ordination.

Start Position

Lying on the mat, place the ball between the ankles, legs straight directly above the hips, feet parallel, softly pointed, arms rested by the sides of the body.

Inhale to prepare and engage the abdominals.

Exhale to curl the upper spine off the mat, nod the head and curl the head, neck then shoulders off the mat, reaching the arms alongside the body, maintain the scapula stability, lower the legs slightly forward.

Inhale to hold the position, keep the ball as still and stable as possible, raise the arms slightly off the mat maintaining the scapula stability.

Exhale for a count of 5 small beats with the arms, inhale for 5 small beats of the arms.

When you have completed 10 sets of inhaling for 5 beats and exhaling for 5 beats.

Inhale to curl the upper body down returning the shoulders, neck and head to the mat, lower the arms to the sides of the body whilst simultaneously raising the legs to above the hips.

Technical Points

Keep the shoulders open and the scapula stabilised.

Maintain the ball as still and stable as possible as the arms are beating at the sides of the body.

Keep the legs straight and ensure the tailbone remains on the mat as the upper body curls forward.

Keep the neck relaxed.

Repetitions

1 Set of The One Hundred with the ball between the ankles.

Contra-indications

Avoid with lower back pain or disc injuries.

Avoid with neck pain or whiplash pathology.

Avoid during pregnancy.

Basic Anatomy

Transversus Abdominus
Oblique Abdominals
Rectus Abdominus
Multifidus
Hamstrings
Quadriceps
Illiopsoas
Deep Neck Flexors
Scapula Stabilisers

p-i-l-a-t-e-s
Stability Ball - Roll Up - Level 4
Exercise 57 - Small Pulses

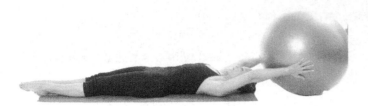

Exercise Focus

This exercise strengthens the abdominals and hip flexors whilst mobilising the spine.

Start Position

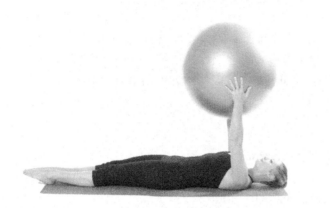

Lying on the mat, legs extended along the floor, legs straight and adducted, feet softly pointed, hold the ball above the shoulders, arms straight, hands to the sides of the ball.

Inhale to prepare and engage the abdominals.

Exhale to nod the head, draw the chin down slightly and curl the head, neck, shoulders and spine off the mat, keep the legs straight and adducted, as the shoulders pass in front of the hips, roll the ball along the legs and over the feet and continue the stretch forwards.

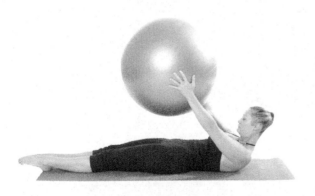

Inhale and stretching the spine forwards, pulse the upper body forwards for 5 small end range pulses.

Exhale to initiate the roll back from the tailbone curling under, continue to roll the spine down sequentially onto the mat, when the ball reaches the knees, raise the ball into the air to challenge the abdominals and continue to roll the spine down, shoulders, neck, head.

Inhale to raise ball slightly backwards behind the head and repeat the roll up.

Technical Points

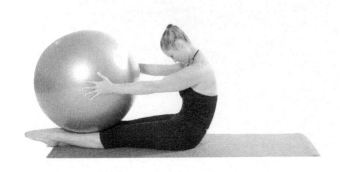

Keep the scapula stabilised throughout the exercise.

Try not to protract the shoulder blades and increase the kyphosis in the thoracic spine on the roll up and down.

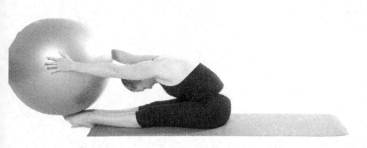

Keep the legs adducted and straight.

Peel each vertebrae off the mat bone by bone, be aware of rolling the spine up and down in one straight line.

Keep the end range pulses small and controlled.

Try not to collapse the upper body onto the legs when stretching forwards, keep the spine lengthening up and over.

Maintain the eye focus on the abdominals when rolling up and down through the spine.

Keep the neck relaxed.

Repetitions

5 Roll Ups with 5 Small Pulses Forward on the Ball.

Contra-indications

Avoid with lower back pain or disc injuries.

Avoid with neck pain or whiplash pathology.

Avoid during pregnancy.

Basic Anatomy

Transversus Abdominus
Oblique Abdominals
Rectus Abdominus
Multifidus
Hamstrings
Adductors
Hip Flexors
Quadriceps
Illiopsoas
Deep Neck Flexors
Scapula Stabilisers

p-i-l-a-t-e-s
Stability Ball - Single Leg Circles - Level 4
Exercise 58 - Pelvis Lifted

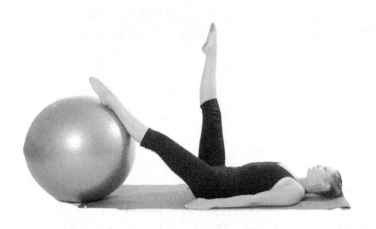

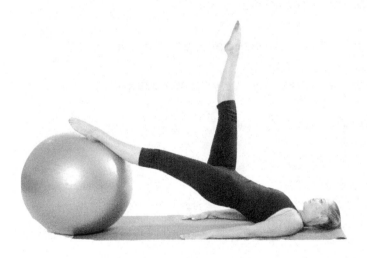

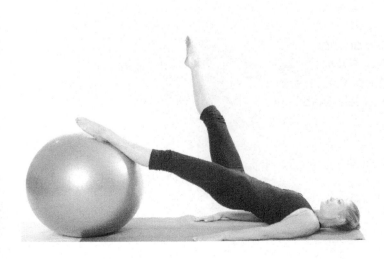

Exercise Focus

This exercise challenges pelvic stability and alignment whilst strengthening the hamstrings, gluteals, quadriceps and hip flexors of the leg.

Start Position

Lying on the mat, place the feet hip width apart, pelvis and spine in a neutral position, arms rested by the sides of the body, place the ball under the right heel.

Inhale to prepare and engage the abdominals.

Exhale to roll the right heel away from the hip until the right leg is straight, raise the left leg into the air as high into the air as possible keeping the tailbone on the mat.

Inhale to engage the abdominals and raise the pelvis off the mat keeping the pelvis level.

Exhale to maintain both legs straight, circle the left leg outwards for 3 small circles, keep the ball still and stable, keep the pelvis lifted.

Inhale to circle the left leg inwards for 3 small circles, inhaling for 3 small circles.

Exhale to lower the left leg down and place the left heel on the ball, keep the pelvis still and lifted.

Inhale to raise the right heel off the ball into the air, raise the right leg as high as possible keeping the pelvis stable.

Inhale as you circle the right leg outwards for 3 small circles, inhaling for 3 circles.

Exhale to circle the right legs inwards for 3 small circles, exhaling for 3 circles.

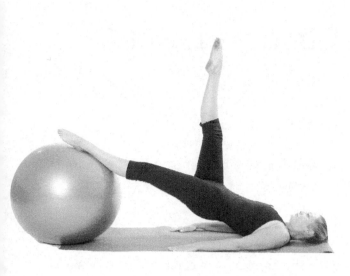

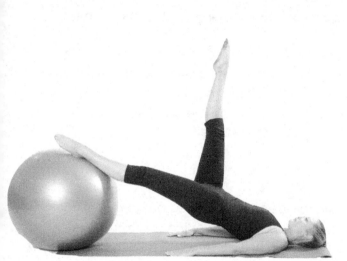

To finish lower the right leg down and place the right heel onto the ball, roll the spine down sequentially bone by bone onto the mat until the pelvis returns to a neutral position.

Technical Points

Keep the shoulders relaxed throughout the exercise.

Maintain the ball as still and stable as possible as the working leg is circling.

Keep the legs straight and ensure the tailbone remains on the mat.

Try not to twist the pelvis to one side as the legs change on the ball.

Try not to hip hike the pelvis during the exercise.

Maintain a still and stable pelvis as the leg circles around.

Repetitions

2 Sets of 3 Leg Circles with the Pelvis Lifted on the Ball.

Contra-indications

Avoid with lower back pain or disc injuries.

Avoid with neck pain or whiplash pathology.

Avoid during pregnancy.

Basic Anatomy

Transversus Abdominus
Oblique Abdominals
Multifidus
Hamstrings
Quadriceps
Illiopsoas
Scapula Stabilisers

p-i-l-a-t-e-s
Stability Ball - Single Leg Stretch - Level 4
Exercise 59 - Twist

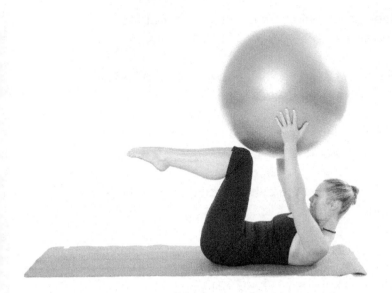

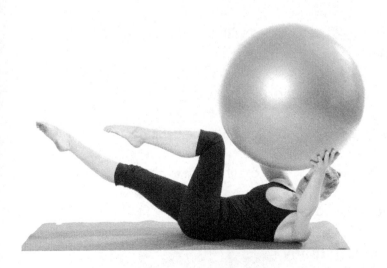

Exercise Focus

This exercise is very challenging for the abdominals and hip flexors.

Start Position

Lying on the semi-supine on the mat, knees and feet hip width apart, pelvis in neutral, place the ball in the hands, arms straight, directly above the shoulders, stabilise the scapula.

Inhale to prepare and engage the abdominals.

Exhale to curl the upper spine forward, draw the chin gently towards the chest, curl the head, neck and shoulders off the mat simultaneously lowering the ball forwards, bring the right leg up to the "table top" position, then the left.

Inhale to hold the position.

Exhale to extend the right leg out to 45° maintain the curl up of the upper spine and rotate the shoulders and head to the left, take the ball over to the left, maintain the arms directly in line with the shoulders.

Inhale to simultaneously bring the right leg in towards the chest, return the right leg to the "table top" position whilst simultaneously extending the left leg away from the hip out to 45°, rotate the upper body to the right rolling onto the right side of the rib cage and shoulder blade, take the ball to the right side, keep the arms in line with the shoulders.

Exhale to simultaneously bring the left leg in towards the chest, return the left leg to the "table top" position, curl towards the left and repeat the exercise.

Technical Points

Maintain the pelvis and spine in neutral as the leg fully extends away from the hip, try not to allow the lumbar lordosis to increase.

Try not to take the ball too far to the side, keep the arms directly in line with the shoulders.

Keep the shoulder blades drawing down the back.

Maintain the eye focus on the abdominals to keep the head on top of the spine.

Keep the navel drawn gently back towards the spine throughout the entire exercise.

Keep both legs parallel.

Try not to posteriorly tilt the pelvis under as the leg draws in towards the body.

Repetitions

10 Single Leg Stretch Twist on the Ball.

Contra-indications

Avoid with lower back pain or disc injuries.

Avoid with neck pain or pathology such as whiplash or osteoarthritis.

Avoid during pregnancy.

Basic Anatomy

Transversus Abdominus
Oblique Abdominals
Rectus Abdominus
Multifidus
Quadriceps
Hip Flexors
Illiopsoas
Scapula Stabilisers
Arm Extensors

p-i-l-a-t-e-s
Stability Ball - Double Leg Stretch - Level 4
Exercise 60 - Hands Up

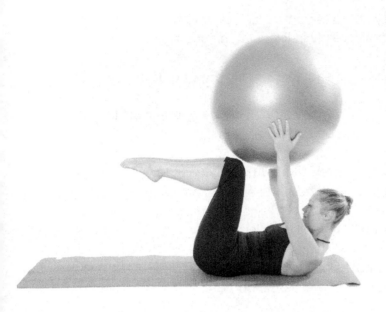

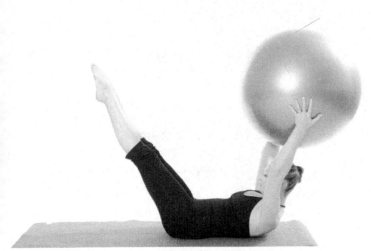

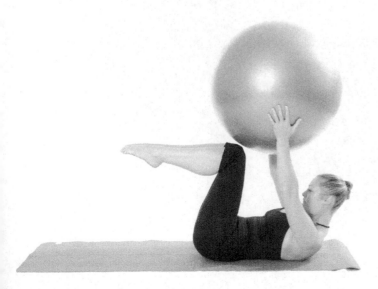

Exercise Focus

This exercise is very challenging for the abdominals, hip flexors and scapula stabilisers.

Start Position

Lying on the semi-supine on the mat, knees and feet hip width apart, pelvis in neutral, place the ball in the hands, arms straight, directly above the shoulders, stabilise the scapula.

Inhale to prepare and engage the abdominals.

Exhale to curl the upper spine forward, draw the chin gently towards the chest, curl the head, neck and shoulders off the mat simultaneously lowering the ball forwards, bring the right leg up to the "table top" position, then the left, legs adducted and parallel.

Inhale to hold the position.

Exhale to extend both legs away from the hip to about 70°, keep the legs adducted and parallel, extend the arms slightly backwards maintaining the upper body curl and scapula stability.

Inhale to bring the arms and legs back towards the body returning to the start position.

Technical Points

Be mindful of the lower back, only take the legs to where the abdominals can be maintained, be careful the lower back doesn't arch away from the mat.

Keep the shoulder blades drawing down the back.

Maintain the eye focus on the abdominals to keep the head on top of the spine.

Keep the navel drawn gently back towards the spine throughout the entire exercise.

Keep both legs parallel and adducted.

Try not to posteriorly tilt the pelvis under as the leg draws in towards the body.

Repetitions

6 Double Leg Stretch Hands Up on the Ball.

Contra-indications

Avoid with lower back pain or disc injuries.

Avoid with neck pain or pathology such as whiplash or osteoarthritis.

Avoid during pregnancy.

Basic Anatomy

Transversus Abdominus
Oblique Abdominals
Rectus Abdominus
Multifidus
Quadriceps
Hip Flexors
Illiopsoas
Adductors
Scapula Stabilisers
Shoulder Extensors

p-i-l-a-t-e-s
Stability Ball - Scissors - Level 4
Exercise 61 - Hands Up

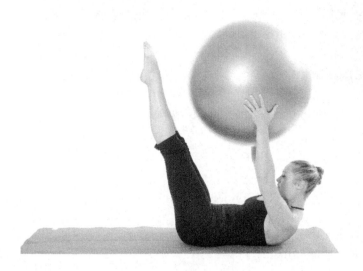

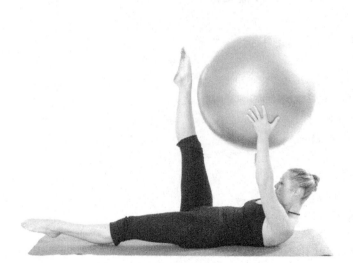

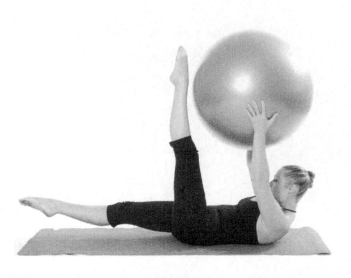

Exercise Focus

This exercise strengthens the hip flexors and abdominals whilst challenging pelvic stability.

Start Position

Lying on the semi-supine on the mat, knees and feet hip width apart, pelvis in neutral, place the ball in the hands, arms straight, directly above the shoulders, stabilise the scapula.

Inhale to prepare and engage the abdominals.

Exhale to curl the upper spine forward, draw the chin gently towards the chest, curl the head, neck and shoulders off the mat simultaneously lowering the ball forwards, bring the right leg up to the "table top" position, then the left, extend both legs towards the ceiling 90° above the hips.

Inhale to hold the position.

Exhale to lower the right leg down towards the floor whilst maintaining the upper body curl.

Inhale to simultaneously bring the right leg up towards the ceiling whilst lowering the left leg straight down towards the floor.

Exhale to simultaneously bring the left leg up towards the ceiling, whilst lowering the right leg down towards the mat and continue the exercise.

Technical Points

Maintain the pelvis and spine in neutral as the leg fully extends away from the hip, try not to allow the lumbar lordosis to increase.

Try not to allow the pelvis to tilt from side to side as the legs lower away from the hip.

Keep the shoulder blades drawing down the back.

Maintain the eye focus on the abdominals to keep the head on top of the spine.

Keep the navel drawn gently back towards the spine throughout the entire exercise.

Keep both legs parallel.

Try not to posteriorly tilt the pelvis under as the leg draws in towards the body.

Repetitions

10 Scissors Hands Up on the Ball.

Contra-indications

Avoid with lower back pain or disc injuries.

Avoid with neck pain or pathology such as whiplash or osteoarthritis.

Avoid during pregnancy.

Basic Anatomy

Transversus Abdominus
Oblique Abdominals
Rectus Abdominus
Multifidus
Quadriceps
Hip Flexors
Illiopsoas
Scapula Stabilisers
Arm Extensors

p-i-l-a-t-e-s
Stability Ball - Side To Side - Level 4
Exercise 62 - Legs Straight

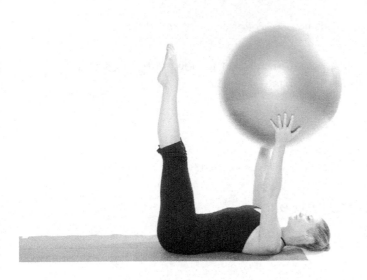

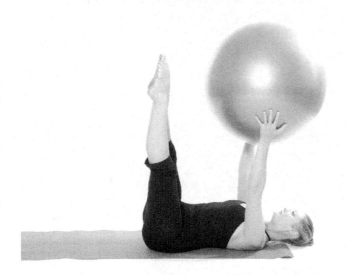

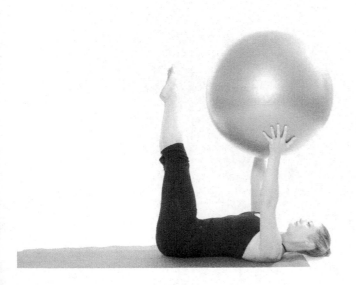

Exercise Focus

This exercise strengthens the oblique abdominals, hip flexors and adductors whilst stretching and strengthening the rotores muscles of the spine.

Start Position

Lying on the semi-supine on the mat, place the ball between the feet, arms are extended towards the ceiling above the shoulders, extend the legs directly above the hips, feet softly pointed.

Inhale to engage the abdominals take both legs over to the right, keep the arms still directly above the shoulders, the rotation is purely from the spine and pelvis, keep the legs straight and adducted.

Exhale to use the abdominals to return the legs to the centre directly above the hips.

Inhale to roll onto the left side of the pelvis, keep the shoulder blades in contact with the mat.

Exhale to use the abdominals and return the legs to the centre.

Technical Points

Keep the shoulder blades in contact with the floor.

Try not to hip hike the pelvis on one side as the legs are taken to the side.

Keep the navel drawn gently back towards the spine throughout the entire exercise.

Keep the opposite shoulder blade in contact with the mat as the legs roll to the side.

Try not to posteriorly tilt the pelvis under as the legs return the ball to the centre.

Repetitions

5 Side to Side with Legs Straight with the Ball.

Contra-indications

Avoid with lower back pain or disc injuries.

Avoid with neck pain or pathology such as whiplash or osteoarthritis.

Avoid during pregnancy.

Basic Anatomy

Transversus Abdominus
Oblique Abdominals
Multifidus
Hip Flexors
Adductors
Spinal Rotores
Scapula Stabilisers
Arm Extensors

p-i-l-a-t-e-s
Stability Ball - Upper Back Lifts - Level 4
Exercise 63 - Arm Circles

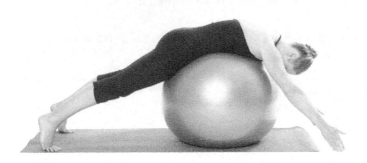

Exercise Focus

This exercise strengthens the spinal extensors and mobilises the shoulder joint.

Start Position

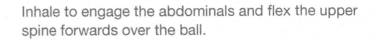

Kneeling on the mat, place the pelvis on the ball, feet are slightly wider than hip width apart, feet parallel, place the ball of the feet against the wall for support, arms reaching over head, scapula stabilised, ensure the body is in one straight line from the head to the feet.

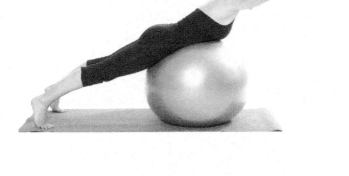

Inhale to engage the abdominals and flex the upper spine forwards over the ball.

Exhale keeping the legs straight, lift the upper back and extend the spine as far back as comfortable, keep the arms straight and in line with the shoulders.

Inhale to reach the arms out to the sides of the body and flex the upper spine forwards and continue to circle the arms down towards the floor as the spine flexes forwards.

Technical Points

Try to work from the mid thoracic muscle region of the back extensors, try not to over use the lumbar back extensors.

Keep the head in line with the spine.

Maintain the scapula stability throughout the entire circle.

Keep the legs straight and use the buttocks.

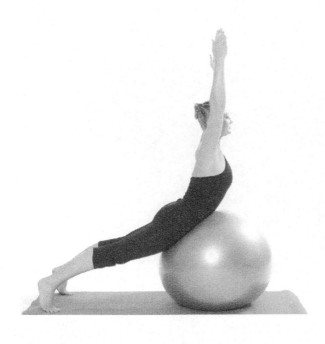

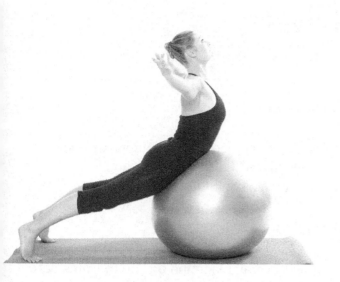

Repetitions

10 Upper Back Lifts with Arm Circles each side on the Ball.

Contra-indications

Avoid with neck pain.

Avoid with lower back pain.

Avoid with shoulder pain or impingement pathology.

Basic Anatomy

Transversus Abdominus
Oblique Abdominals
Multifidus
Erector Spinae
Middle and Lower Trapezius
Hamstrings
Gluteus Maximus
Arm Extensors

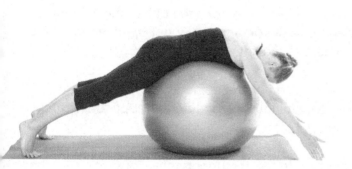

p-i-l-a-t-e-s
Stability Ball - Side Lifts - Level 4
Exercise 64 - Twist

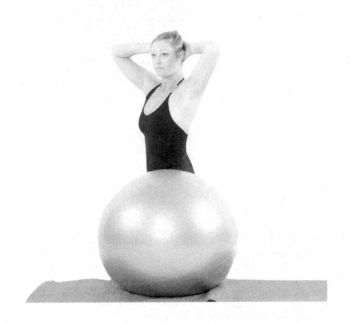

Exercise Focus

This exercise strengthens and stretches the side flexors of the spine, it also stretches and strengthens the spinal rotators of the thoracic.

Start Position

Kneeling on the mat, place the ball on the left side of the body, place the hip left hip on the ball, feet are slightly wider than hip width apart, left foot in front, right foot on the ball of the foot, hands interlaced behind the head, scapula stabilised, ensure the body is in one straight line from the head to the hip.

Inhale to engage the abdominals and side flex the upper spine forwards over the ball to the left whilst simultaneously rotating the upper spine and shoulders to the left.

Exhale to side flex the spine towards the right hip, whilst simultaneously rotating the upper spine and shoulders to the right.

Inhale to side flex the upper spine forwards over the ball to the left whilst rotating the upper spine and shoulders to the left and continue the exercise.

Technical Points

Keep the ball stable throughout the exercise.

Keep the movement flowing.

Try not to rotate the shoulders forwards on the side flexion.

Keep the pelvis stable, try not to rotate the pelvis backwards.

Repetitions

10 Side Lifts with Twist on the Ball.

Contra-indications

Avoid with neck pain.

Avoid with lower back pain.

Avoid with shoulder pain or impingement pathology.

Basic Anatomy

Transversus Abdominus
Oblique Abdominals
Multifidus
Erector Spinae
Paraspinals
Quadratus Lumborum
Middle and Lower Trapezius
Hamstrings
Adductors
Gluteus Maximus
Arm Extensors

p-i-l-a-t-e-s
Stability Ball - Side Leg Series - Level 4
Exercise 65 - Bicycle

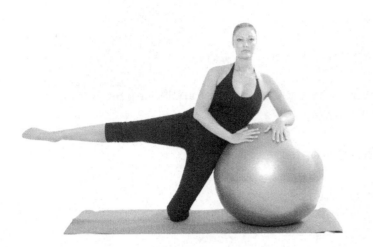

Exercise Focus

This exercise strengthens the muscles of the hip and leg whilst challenging core and pelvic stability.

Start Position

Place the ball on the left side of the body, lean the left hip onto the ball and place the left elbow on top of the ball, extend the right leg directly to the side, right foot pointed, place the right hand on the ball for stability, do not collapse into the shoulders.

Inhale to prepare and engage the abdominals.

Exhale to raise the right leg off the floor keeping the upper body still.

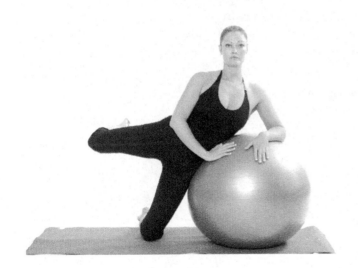

Inhale to bend the right knee taking the right foot behind the hip, keep inhaling whilst flexing the right leg at the hip bringing the knee forwards of the hip.

Exhale to extend the right leg forwards to fully straighten the leg, keep the leg parallel and lifted as high as possible.

Inhale to sweep the right leg behind the hip and continue the exercise.

Change sides and repeat the exercise.

Technical Points

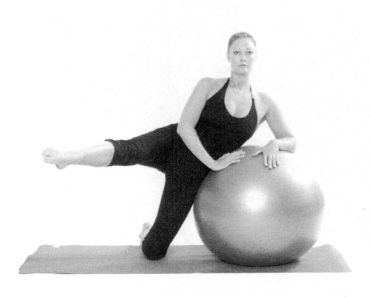

Keep the body still on the ball as the leg sweeps forward and back.

Try not to roll the ball forwards and backwards, keep as stable as possible.

Maintain the scapula stability when resting the upper body on the ball.

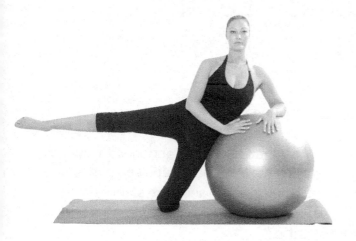

Keep the pelvis still as the leg lifts and lowers, isolate the movement in the hip abductors.

Repetitions

10 Side Leg Lifts Bicycle on the Ball.

Contra-indications

Avoid with neck pain.

Avoid with lower back pain.

Avoid with shoulder pain or impingement pathology.

Basic Anatomy

Transversus Abdominus
Oblique Abdominals
Multifidus
Erector Spinae
Paraspinals
Quadratus Lumborum
Abductors of the Hip
Hamstrings

p-i-l-a-t-e-s
Stability Ball - Knee Stretches - Level 4
Exercise 66 - Knees Lifted

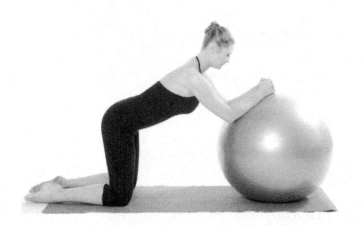

Exercise Focus

This exercise strengthens the abdominals, scapula stabilisers, hip flexors, quadriceps and hamstrings whilst challenging pelvic and core stability.

Start Position

Kneeling on the mat, feet and knees hip width apart, place the ball in front of the body, place the elbows and forearms resting on the top of the ball, spine and pelvis in neutral, stabilise the shoulders down the back, keep the head in line with the spine.

Inhale to prepare and engage the abdominals.

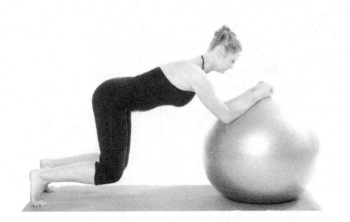

Exhale to raise the knees just off the mat maintaining the neutral spine and pelvis.

Inhale to slowly roll the ball forwards keeping the knees lifted off the mat.

Exhale to slowly roll the ball in towards the hips, maintain the neutral spine and pelvis.

Inhale to roll the ball forwards and repeat the exercise.

Technical Points

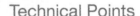

Try not to arch the lower back as the ball rolls forwards and backwards, maintain a neutral spine.

Keep control of the ball in both directions.

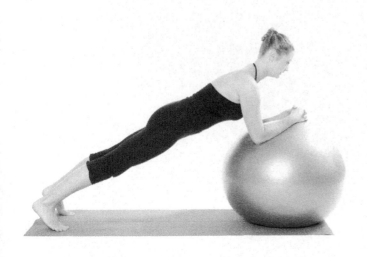

Try not to collapse the upper thoracic spine and bring the scapula together.

Keep the shoulders drawn down the back and head in line with the spine.

Repetitions

10 Knee Stretches with Knees Lifted on the Ball.

Contra-indications

Avoid with neck pain.

Avoid with lower back pain.

Avoid with shoulder pain or impingement pathology.

Basic Anatomy

Transversus Abdominus
Oblique Abdominals
Multifidus
Erector Spinae
Hip Flexors
Quadriceps
Hamstrings
Serratus Anterior
Rhomboids
Latissimus Dorsi
Middle and Lower Trapezius
Pectorals

p-i-l-a-t-e-s
Stability Ball - Leg Pull Back - Level 4
Exercise 67 - Pelvic Lift

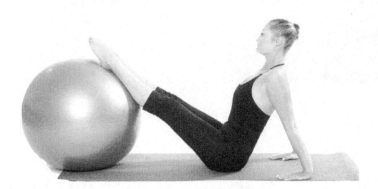

Exercise Focus

This exercise is very challenging for the hamstrings and gluteals.

Start Position

Sitting on the mat, legs extended in front of the body, place the ball under the heels/mid calves, legs adducted, feet pointed, hands placed on the mat slightly behind the shoulder joint, fingers facing forward, arms straight, elbows soft, stabilise the scapula.

Inhale to prepare.

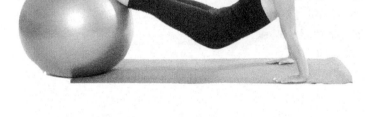

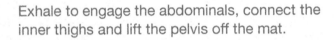

Exhale to engage the abdominals, connect the inner thighs and lift the pelvis off the mat.

Inhale to slowly lower the pelvis onto the mat with control.

Exhale to raise the pelvis off the mat, maintain the legs straight and continue the exercise.

Technical Points

Try not to collapse between the shoulder blades or allow the shoulders to elevate into the neck.

Keep the elbows soft.

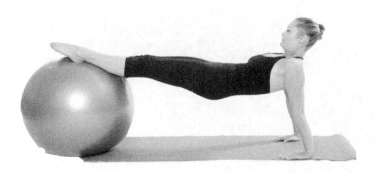

If the client finds this exercise too difficult for the wrists, turn the hands to face the fingers to the side, but not behind.

If the client finds this exercise too difficult with legs straight, bend the knees and place the ball closer to the body under the knee joints.

Try not to arch the back when lifting the pelvis.

Keep the eyes focused forward try not to look up to the ceiling when lifting the pelvis.

Repetitions

4 Pelvic Lifts with Straight Legs on the Ball.

Contra-indications

Avoid with neck pain.

Avoid with lower back pain.

Avoid with shoulder pain or impingement pathology.

Avoid with wrist pain.

Avoid with knee pain or knee instability.

Basic Anatomy

Transversus Abdominus
Oblique Abdominals
Multifidus
Erector Spinae
Hamstrings
Gluteals
Serratus Posterior
Rhomboids
Latissimus Dorsi
Middle and Lower Trapezius

p-i-l-a-t-e-s
Core Stability Ball - Roll Over - Level 5
Exercise 68 - Ball Between Ankles

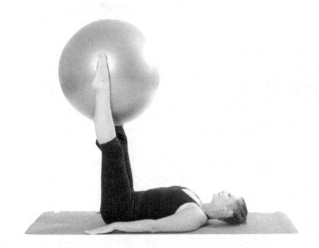

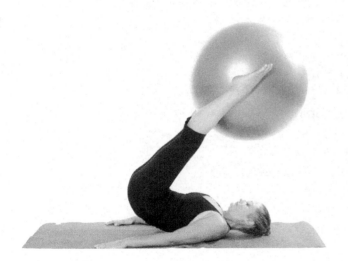

Exercise Focus

This exercise stretches the spine and hamstrings whilst strengthening the abdominals and adductors.

Start Position

Lying on the mat, place the ball between the ankles, legs straight directly above the hips, feet parallel, softly pointed, arms rested by the sides of the body.

Inhale to prepare and engage the abdominals.

Exhale to initiate the roll over from curling the tailbone under and posteriorly tilting the pelvis, roll the spine over taking the ball over the head.

Inhale to hold the position, lightly squeeze the ball using the adductors.

Exhale to roll the spine back onto the mat sequentially and with control.

Inhale to hold the legs at 90° and prepare to roll over again.

Technical Points

Keep the shoulders open and the scapula stabilised.

Keep the movement flowing and controlled.

When taking the legs and ball over the head try not to touch the ball or feet to the floor, maintain the legs parallel to the floor.

Keep the knees straight.

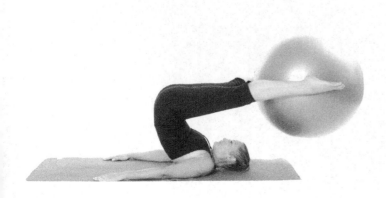

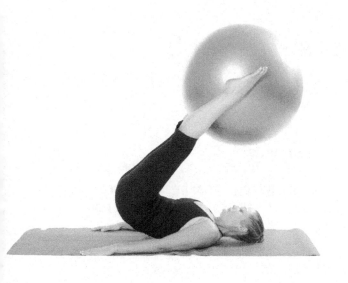

Try not to over use the arms in controlling the movement, focus on controlling from the abdominals.

Keep the neck relaxed.

Repetitions

4 Roll Overs with the Ball.

Contra-indications

Avoid with lower back pain or disc injuries.

Avoid with neck pain or whiplash pathology.

Avoid during pregnancy.

Basic Anatomy

Transversus Abdominus
Oblique Abdominals
Rectus Abdominus
Multifidus
Adductors
Quadriceps
Illiopsoas
Hip Flexors
Deep Neck Flexors
Scapula Stabilisers

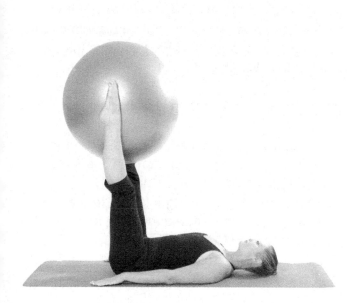

p-i-l-a-t-e-s
Core Stability Ball - Scissors - Level 5
Exercise 69 - Twist

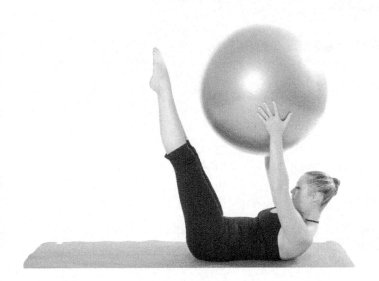

Exercise Focus

This exercise strengthens the hip flexors and oblique abdominals whilst challenging pelvic stability.

Start Position

Lying on the semi-supine on the mat, knees and feet hip width apart, pelvis in neutral, place the ball in the hands, arms straight, directly above the shoulders, stabilise the scapula.

Inhale to prepare and engage the abdominals.

Exhale to curl the upper spine forward, draw the chin gently towards the chest, curl the head, neck and shoulders off the mat simultaneously lowering the ball forwards, bring the right leg up to the "table top" position, then the left, extend both legs towards the ceiling 90° above the hips.

Inhale to hold the position.

Exhale to lower the right leg down towards the floor whilst curling the upper body, shoulders and head towards the left leg, take the arms to the side, keep the arms in line with the shoulders.

Inhale to simultaneously bring the right leg up towards the ceiling whilst lowering the left leg straight down towards the floor, curl the upper body to the right taking the ball to the right side, keep the arms directly in line with the shoulders.

Exhale to simultaneously bring the left leg up towards the ceiling, whilst lowering the right leg down towards the mat and continue the exercise.

Technical Points

Maintain the pelvis and spine in neutral as the leg fully extends away from the hip, try not to allow the lumbar lordosis to increase.

Try not to rotate the upper body too far, keep the rotation small and controlled.

Try not to allow the pelvis to tilt from side to side as the legs lower away from the hip.

Keep the shoulder blades drawing down the back.

Maintain the eye focus on the abdominals to keep the head on top of the spine.

Keep the navel drawn gently back towards the spine throughout the entire exercise.

Keep both legs parallel.

Try not to posteriorly tilt the pelvis under as the leg draws in towards the body.

Repetitions

10 Scissors with Twist on the Ball.

Contra-indications

Avoid with lower back pain or disc injuries.

Avoid with neck pain or pathology such as whiplash or osteoarthritis.

Avoid during pregnancy.

Basic Anatomy

Transversus Abdominus
Oblique Abdominals
Rectus Abdominus
Multifidus
Quadriceps
Hip Flexors
Illiopsoas
Scapula Stabilisers
Arm Extensors

p-i-l-a-t-e-s
Core Stability Ball - Upper Back Lifts - Level 5
Exercise 70 - Rotation

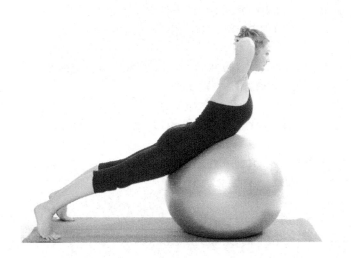

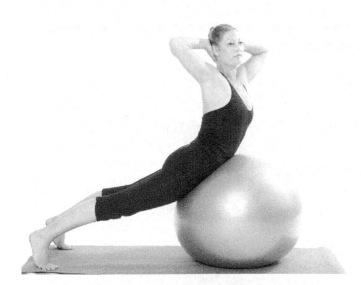

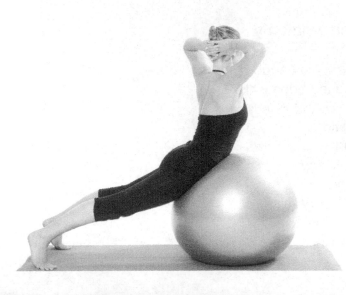

Exercise Focus

This exercise strengthens the spinal extensors and thoracic spine.

Start Position

Kneeling on the mat, place the pelvis on the ball, feet are slightly wider than hip width apart, feet parallel, place the ball of the feet against the wall for support, interlace the hands behind the head, scapula stabilised, ensure the body is in one straight line from the head to the feet.

Inhale to engage the abdominals and flex the upper spine forwards over the ball.

Exhale keeping the legs straight, lift the upper back and extend the spine as far back as comfortable, keep the elbows open and scapula stabilised.

Inhale to rotate the shoulders and upper body to the right.

Exhale to rotate the spine and shoulders to the centre.

Inhale to rotate the shoulders and upper body to the left.

Exhale to return the head, shoulders and upper spine to the centre.

Inhale to flex the upper spine forwards over the ball.

Technical Points

Try to work from the mid thoracic muscle region of the back extensors, try not to over use the lumbar back extensors.

Try not to raise the shoulders as the spine rotates from one side to the other.

Keep the head in line with the spine.

Maintain the scapula stability throughout the entire circle.

Keep the legs straight and use the buttocks.

Repetitions

10 Upper Back Lifts with Rotation each side on the Ball.

Contra-indications

Avoid with neck pain.

Avoid with lower back pain.

Avoid with shoulder pain or impingement pathology.

Basic Anatomy

Transversus Abdominus
Oblique Abdominals
Multifidus
Erector Spinae
Middle and Lower Trapezius
Hamstrings
Gluteus Maximus
Arm Extensors

p-i-l-a-t-e-s
Core Stability Ball - Leg Pull Back - Level 5
Exercise 71 - Lift Leg

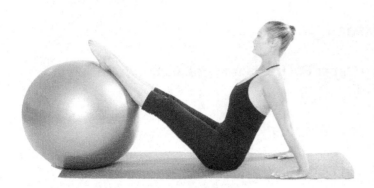

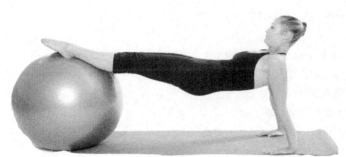

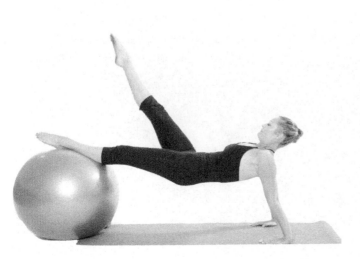

Exercise Focus

This exercise is very challenging for the hamstrings, gluteals and upper body.

Start Position

Sitting on the mat, legs extended in front of the body, place the ball under the heels/mid calves, legs adducted, feet pointed, hands placed on the mat slightly behind the shoulder joint, fingers facing forward, arms straight, elbows soft, stabilise the scapula.

Inhale to prepare.

Exhale to engage the abdominals, connect the inner thighs and lift the pelvis off the mat.

Inhale to hold the position.

Exhale to raise the right foot just off the ball.

Inhale to lower the right foot to the ball.

Exhale to lift the left foot just off the ball.

Inhale to lower the left foot to the ball.

Exhale to hold the position.

Inhale to slowly lower the pelvis onto the mat with control.

Exhale to raise the pelvis off the mat, maintain the legs straight and continue the exercise.

Technical Points

Try not to collapse between the shoulder blades or allow the shoulders to elevate into the neck.

If the client finds this exercise too difficult fo wrists, turn the hands to face the fingers to the side, but not behind.

If the client finds this exercise too difficult with legs straight, bend the knees and place the ball closer to the body under the knee joints.

Try not to arch the back when lifting the pelvis.

Keep the eyes focused forward try not to look up to the ceiling when lifting the pelvis.

Repetitions

2 Pelvic Lifts with Leg Lifts on the Ball.

Contra-indications

Avoid with neck pain.

Avoid with lower back pain.

Avoid with shoulder pain or impingement pathology.

Avoid with wrist pain.

Avoid with knee pain or knee instability.

Basic Anatomy

Transversus Abdominus
Oblique Abdominals
Multifidus
Erector Spinae
Hamstrings
Gluteals
Serratus Posterior
Rhomboids
Latissimus Dorsi
Middle and Lower Trapezius

p-i-l-a-t-e-s
Core Stability Ball - Leg Pull Front - Level 5
Exercise 72 - Lift Leg

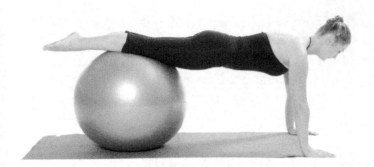

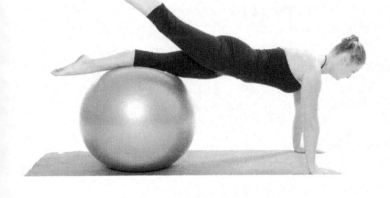

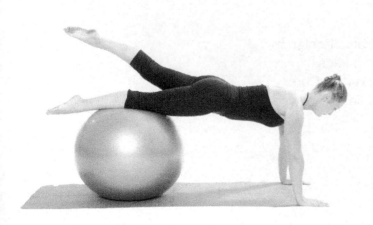

Exercise Focus

This exercise challenges core and pelvic stability and strengthens the scapula stabilisers, hamstrings and gluteals.

Start Position

Kneeling on the mat, place the body on the ball and roll the body forwards on the ball until the mid-thighs and knees are placed on the ball, take the arms slightly wider than shoulder width apart, stabilise the scapula.

Inhale to prepare and engage the abdominals.

Exhale to raise the right leg off the ball behind the right hip, keep the legs straight.

Inhale to lower the right leg back to the ball.

Exhale to lift the left leg off the ball.

Inhale to lower the left leg back onto the ball.

Exhale bend the knees and press through the arms, roll the ball back until the feet touch the floor and dismount the ball with control.

Technical Points

Keep the spine and pelvis in neutral.

Try not to poke the head forward as the leg lifts.

Keep the spine lengthened.

Try not to collapse the shoulder blades together, keep the scapula still and isolate the press in and out from the arms only.

Keep the abdominals gently drawn back towards the spine.

Ensure the weight is evenly distributed on both arms.

Repetitions

3 Sets of Leg Pull Front on the Ball.

Contra-indications

Avoid with shoulder pain.

Avoid with shoulder impingement pain.

Avoid with tight pectorals or upper crossed syndrome postural types.

Avoid with lower back pain.

Avoid with osteoporosis or kyphotic postural types.

Basic Anatomy

Transversus Abdominus
Oblique Abdominals
Multifidus
Erector Spinae
Pectorals Major and Minor
Anterior Deltoid
Serratus Anterior
Rhomboids
Middle and Lower Trapezius
Biceps
Triceps
Wrist Extensors
Arm Flexors and Extensors

p-i-l-a-t-e-s
Core Stability Ball - Knee Pull In - Level 5
Exercise 73 - Knees In/Out

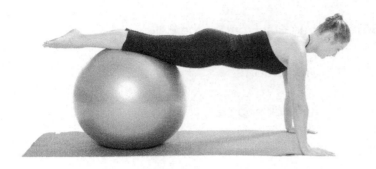

Exercise Focus

This exercise challenges core and pelvic stability and strengthens the scapula stabilisers and hip flexors.

Start Position

Kneeling on the mat, place the body on the ball and roll the body forwards on the ball until the mid-thighs and knees are placed on the ball, take the arms slightly wider than shoulder width apart, stabilise the scapula.

Inhale to prepare and engage the abdominals.

Exhale to draw both knees in towards the chest, keep the legs together and parallel and allow the ball to roll in towards the hands.

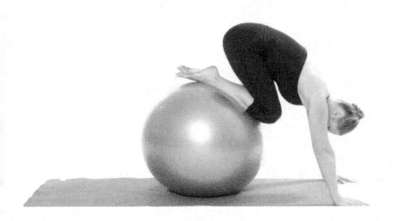

Inhale to slowly roll the ball away from the hands with control until both legs are fully straightened.

Repeat the knee pull in 6 times then,

Exhale press through the arms, roll the ball back until the feet touch the floor and dismount the ball with control.

Technical Points

Keep the spine and pelvis in neutral.

Keep the spine lengthened.

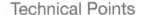

Try not to drop the lower back when extending the legs away from the hips.

Try not to collapse the shoulder blades together, keep the scapula still and isolate the press in and out from the arms only.

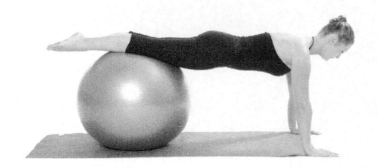

Visualise a strip of tape along the mat, roll the ball along the line.

Keep the abdominals gently drawn back towards the spine.

Ensure the weight is evenly distributed on both arms.

Repetitions

2 Sets of 6 Knee Pull In on the Ball.

Contra-indications

Avoid with shoulder pain.

Avoid with shoulder impingement pain.

Avoid with tight pectorals or upper crossed syndrome postural types.

Avoid with lower back pain.

Avoid with osteoporosis or kyphotic postural types.

Basic Anatomy

Transversus Abdominus
Oblique Abdominals
Multifidus
Erector Spinae
Hip Flexors
Adductors
Illiopsoas
Pectorals Major and Minor
Anterior Deltoid
Serratus Anterior
Rhomboids
Middle and Lower Trapezius
Wrist Extensors

p-i-l-a-t-e-s
Core Stability Ball - Scissor - Level 5
Exercise 74 - Scissor Legs

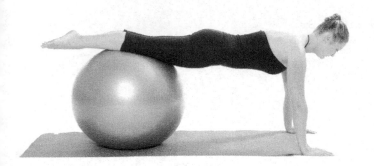

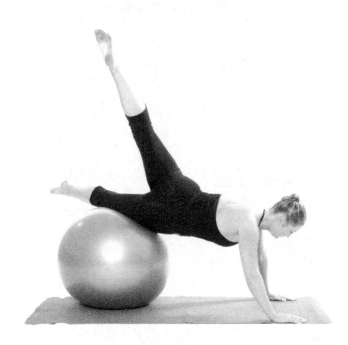

Exercise Focus

A very challenging exercise requiring core stability, balance, control and co-ordination.

Start Position

Kneeling on the mat, place the body on the ball and roll the body forwards on the ball until the mid-thighs and knees are placed on the ball, take the arms slightly wider than shoulder width apart, stabilise the scapula.

Inhale to prepare and engage the abdominals.

Exhale to roll the ball underneath the body to the left whilst simultaneously twisting the body to the right, separating the legs into a wide scissor movement.

Inhale to slowly roll the ball back to the centre whilst simultaneously returning the legs and body to centre on the ball.

Exhale to roll the ball to the right whilst simultaneously twisting the hips to roll the ball under the left hip, separate the legs into a wide scissor position.

Inhale to return the legs and body to the centre and repeat the exercise.

Exhale press through the arms, roll the ball back until the feet touch the floor and dismount the ball with control.

Technical Points

Keep the spine and pelvis in neutral.

Keep the spine lengthened.

Try not to drop the lower back when extending the legs away from the hips.

Try not to collapse the shoulder blades together, keep the scapula still and isolate the press in and out from the arms only.

Visualise a strip of tape along the mat, roll the ball along the line.

Keep the abdominals gently drawn back towards the spine.

Ensure the weight is evenly distributed on both arms.

Repetitions

2 Sets of 2 Scissors each side on the Ball.

Contra-indications

Avoid with shoulder pain.

Avoid with shoulder impingement pain.

Avoid with thoracic pain.

Avoid with tight pectorals or upper crossed syndrome postural types.

Avoid with lower back pain.

Avoid with osteoporosis or kyphotic postural types.

Basic Anatomy

Transversus Abdominus
Oblique Abdominals
Multifidus
Erector Spinae
Adductors
Illiopsoas
Pectorals Major and Minor
Serratus Anterior
Rhomboids
Middle and Lower Trapezius
Wrist Extensors

p-i-l-a-t-e-s
Core Stability Ball - Swan - Level 5
Exercise 75 - Small Push Back

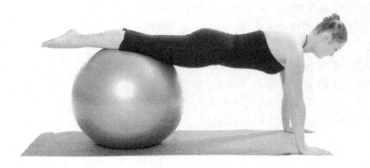

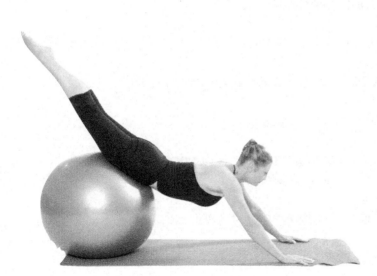

Exercise Focus

This exercise strengthens the back extensors and arms.

Start Position

Kneeling on the mat, place the body on the ball and roll the body forwards on the ball until the mid-thighs and knees are placed on the ball, legs straight and parallel, adducted, take the arms slightly wider than shoulder width apart, stabilise the scapula.

Inhale to prepare and engage the abdominals.

Exhale to press through the arms to roll the ball backwards whilst simultaneously taking the legs up into the air behind the hips.

Inhale to slowly roll the ball forwards allowing the legs to lower and returning to the start position.

Repeat the Swan movement 5 times then,

Exhale press through the arms, roll the ball back until the feet touch the floor and dismount the ball with control.

Technical Points

Keep the spine and pelvis in neutral.

Keep the spine lengthened.

Try not to drop the lower back when extending the legs away from the hips.

Try not to collapse the shoulder blades together, keep the scapula still and isolate the press in and out from the arms only.

Visualise a strip of tape along the mat, roll the ball along the line.

Keep both legs straight and adducted.

Keep the abdominals gently drawn back towards the spine.

Ensure the weight is evenly distributed on both arms.

Repetitions

2 Sets of 5 Swan on the Ball.

Contra-indications

Avoid with shoulder pain.

Avoid with shoulder impingement pain.

Avoid with tight pectorals or upper crossed syndrome postural types.

Avoid with lower back pain.

Avoid with osteoporosis or kyphotic postural types.

Basic Anatomy

Transversus Abdominus
Oblique Abdominals
Multifidus
Erector Spinae
HIp Flexors
Adductors
Illiopsoas
Pectorals Major and Minor
Anterior Deltoid
Serratus Anterior
Rhomboids
Middle and Lower Trapezius
Wrist Extensors

p-i-l-a-t-e-s
Stability Ball - Push Up - Level 5
Exercise 76 - Plank Position

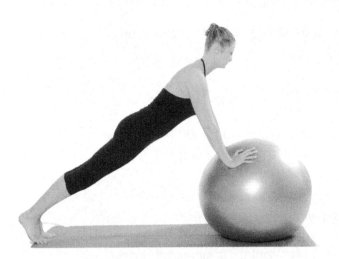

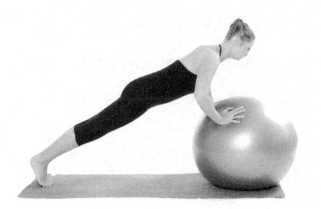

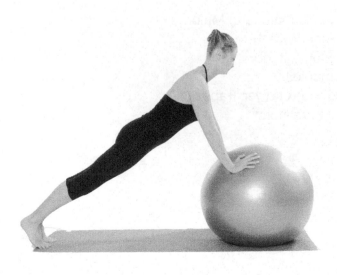

Exercise Focus

This exercise challenges core and pelvic stability and strengthens the scapula stabilisers, pectorals and arm flexors and extensors.

Start Position

Kneeling on the mat, place the hands on the ball in front of the body, ball in line with the shoulders, place the hands on the ball, shoulder width apart, knees and feet together, adducted in parallel.

Inhale to engage the abdominals, slide the right foot behind the hip and take the weight onto the ball of the right foot.

Exhale to slide the left foot behind the left hip and take the weight onto the ball of the left foot.

Inhale to bend the elbows to the side of the body and control the body as it moves closer to the ball, maintain the scapula stability.

Exhale to press the body away from the wall and straighten the arms, keep the shoulders down the back, keep the ball as stable as possible, the spine and pelvis remain in neutral.

Technical Points

Keep the spine and pelvis in neutral.

Try not to poke the head forward as the arms bend.

Keep the spine lengthened.

Try not to collapse the shoulder blades together, keep the scapula still and isolate the press in and out from the arms only.

Keep the abdominals gently drawn back towards the spine.

Ensure the weight is evenly distributed on both arms.

Keep the heels in contact with the floor and the legs straight on the push up.

Repetitions

10 Push Up Plank Position on the Ball.

Contra-indications

Avoid with shoulder pain.

Avoid with shoulder impingement pain.

Avoid with tight pectorals or upper crossed syndrome postural types.

Avoid with osteoporosis or kyphotic postural types.

Basic Anatomy

Transversus Abdominus
Oblique Abdominals
Multifidus
Erector Spinae
Pectorals Major and Minor
Anterior Deltoid
Serratus Anterior
Rhomboids
Middle and Lower Trapezius
Biceps
Triceps
Wrist Extensors
Arm Flexors and Extensors

Legal Notice

Your use of this web site hosted by p-i-l-a-t-e-s PTY LTD and/or its various affiliates or subsidiaries (collectively referred to as 'pilates" is subject to the following terms and conditions:

Disclaimers

Obtain medical clearance from your health care practitioner prior to beginning the exercise programmes described on the site or in the Manuals. The exercises described on this site are not suitable for everyone and are not a substitute for medical expertise. If done improperly, exercise has some risk of injury. If you feel discomfort or pain, DO NOT continue. p-i-l-a-t-e-s PTY LTD disclaim any liability or loss in connection with the exercises described herein.

p-i-l-a-t-e-s PTY LTD makes no warranties or representations of any kind concerning the accuracy or suitability of the information contained on this web site for any purpose. All such information is provided "as is" and with specific disclaimer of any warranties of merchantability, fitness for purpose, title and/or non-infringement. p-i-l-a-t-e-s PTY LTD makes no warranties or representations of any kind that the services provided by this web site will be uninterrupted, error- free or that the web site or the server that hosts the web site are free from viruses or other forms of harmful computer code. In no event shall p-i-l-a-t-e-s PTY LTD, its employees or agents be liable for any direct, indirect or consequential damages resulting from the use of this web site. This exclusion and limitation only applies to the extent permitted by law and is without prejudice to any express provisions to the contrary in any written licence or subscription agreement from p-i-l-a-t-e-s PTY LTD in respect of the use of any online service provided via this web site.

Caution

On standing and kneeling exercises, work with a partner until you have mastered the balance these exercises require.

Privacy

p-i-l-a-t-e-s PTY LTD is committed to protecting your privacy online. Our policy explains how we will do this.

Copyright

What information do we collect?

• We collect email addresses.

 Registration: on some parts of the site may ask you to register, and if you do we may ask for
your name, email address, geographical address and other personal information. From time to time we may ask you for further information, for example if you make a
purchase. We may also use cookies. For an explanation, see the section on cookies below.

How do we use your information?

We use the information to help us understand more about how our web site is used, to improve our site, and to send you information about us and our products which we think may be of interest to you, both electronically or otherwise. Unless you have informed us that you do not wish to receive further information about our products and services and those of our affiliates and partners, we and they may send you direct mail.

When do we share information?

We do not sell your personal information to others.

We share your information with our associated companies, including p-i-l-a-t-e-s PTY LTD internationally. A number of other people's web sites have links on our site. If you link to their sites, they may collect information. Such sites are not within our control and are not covered by this privacy statement. If we believe that your use of the site is unlawful or damaging to others, we reserve the right to disclose the information we have obtained through the site about you to the extent that it is reasonably necessary in our opinion to prevent, remedy or take action in relation to such conduct.

Security

All personal and credit card information is encoded using Secure Sockets Layer (SSL) technology before being sent over the Internet. To protect your data further, your credit card information is always stored in encrypted form in a database that is away from our Web site database, so it isn't connected to the Internet. Credit card transactions are issued a digital certificate, ensuring that your data can only be read by our transaction system as long as your browser shows its secure mode symbol (such as a key or closed lock). To make the most of the security on our site, we recommend using either Netscape Navigator® or Microsoft® Internet ExplorerTM version 4.0 or higher, both of which enable SSL. We also recommend setting your browser's preferences to accept cookies and enable JavaScriptTM.

Use of Cookies

Cookies are small files which many web sites transfer to your hard disk. They can inform the web site what pages you visit, and your preferences, which enable web sites to provide you with a more personalized service. You can set your browser to refuse cookies, or to warn you before accepting them.

We use cookies, but most parts of our site can be accessed even if your cookies are turned off. But you may find there are parts of the site which you cannot access if your cookies are turned off.

Links

Links to other web sites are provided by p-i-l-a-t-e-s PTY LTD in good faith and for information only. p-i-l-a-t-e-s PTY LTD disclaims any responsibility for the materials contained in any web site linked to this site.

Interactive material

Portions of this site may allow users to post their own material. Materials posted by users do not necessarily reflect the views of p-i-l-a-t-e-s PTY LTD. By posting materials on this site, you represent that you have all necessary rights in and to such materials and that such materials will not infringe any personal or proprietary rights of any third parties, nor will such materials be defamatory, unlawful, threatening, obscene or otherwise objectionable. p-i-l-a-t-e-s PTY LTD reserves the right, at its sole discretion, to review, edit or delete any material posted by users which p-i-l-a-t-e-s PTY LTD deems defamatory, unlawful, threatening, obscene or otherwise objectionable. Notwithstanding the foregoing, p-i-l-a-t-e-s PTY LTD expressly disclaims any responsibility or liability for any material communicated by third parties through this web site.

We will review this policy in the light of comments we receive so please check the latest version. If you have any questions specifically about Privacy please contact us.

CPSIA information can be obtained
at www.ICGtesting.com
Printed in the USA
LVOW03s2349011216

515432LV00005B/29/P